D1035280

Discharge Planning for Continuity of Care

New Edition, Expanded and Revised

Evelyn G. Hartigan and D. Jean Brown, Editors

Pub. No. 20-1977

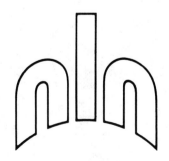

National League for Nursing • New York

12/20/85

Copyright © 1985, 1976 by
National League for Nursing

ISBN 0-88737-160-4

All rights reserved. No part of this book may be
reproduced in print, or by photostatic means, or in
any other manner, without the express written
permission of the publisher.

Manufactured in the United States of America

preface

This book is a greatly revised edition of a work originally published by the National League for Nursing in 1976, *Discharge Planning for Continuity of Care,* which was considered by many health care professionals to be the indispensable guide to the field. Although the first edition still contained some useful information, it needed to be brought up to date and revised to reflect the many recent changes in health care. The present edition expands and elaborates on the material in the first edition, and adds new illustrations, new statistical information, and new analyses of current trends.

The text of the manual consists of three parts. The introduction, Part I, surveys the recent changes in the health care delivery system that have made discharge planning such a pressing concern for health professionals. Part II, The Basics of Discharge Planning, sets out the components of the discharge planning process. It is intended for newcomers to the field as well as for experienced discharge planners.

Part III is a collection of essays that provide more advanced views of discharge planning by those active in the field, including educators and physicians, and a statistical profile of today's discharge planner. Most of the papers in Part III were presented at a series of workshops presented by the Southern Regional Assembly of Constituent Leagues for Nursing and the Georgia, Florida, South Louisiana, and Tennessee Leagues for Nursing in the autumn of 1984.

The appendixes, newly created for this edition, provide much useful information for the experienced or neophyte discharge planner. Appendix A is a compendium of statistical information that will help the reader put the current situation in perspective. Appendix B is a glossary of troublesome names and terms. Appendix C is a compilation of source documents, forms, job descriptions, and evaluation tools that will be of assistance to those who are setting up a new program or evaluating an existing one. In addition, the book contains an extensive bibliography, a list of journals and audiovisual aids, and a list of professional organizations of interest to the discharge planner.

Acknowledgments

Many colleagues gave us advice and helped in the editing of this publication, but the following gave "above and beyond," both in expertise and time: the authors of the first edition, Opal Bristow, Carol Stickney, and Shirley Thompson; Evelyn McNamara and Jo Keblusek for their chapter contributions; Mara Freimanis for the awesome task of gathering the sources for the bibliography; Sarah Craig for the introduction, for sharing many items of information, and for always being available by phone; and Drs. James McNamara and Harold Smith of the University of Utah Health Sciences Center, for sharing their unpublished work with us.

A special thank you to Catherine Olson, librarian, Governors State University; the reference personnel of the American Hospital Association; our typist, Mary Brown; Denise Novoselski of Miramar Publishing Company and the publishers for making available for our use their *Resource Guide* (no longer in print), which aided us in providing a comprehensive reference directory of associations, informative sources, government sources, and charitable organizations, to name a few. Lastly, thank you, Elaine Silverstein, our editor.

Evelyn G. Hartigan
D. Jean Brown

contents

about the contributors

Ruth C. Baker, RN (Chapter 13), is discharge planning coordinator at Tulane Medical Center, New Orleans, Louisiana.

Barbara E. Brown, EdD, RN (Chapter 11), is director of the center for continuing education, Vanderbilt University School of Nursing, Nashville, Tennessee.

D. Jean Brown, BHSN, RN (coeditor; chapters 2, 3, 4, 6, and 7), is a graduate student at Governors State University, University Park, Illinois.

Lynda N. Brown, EdD, RN (Chapter 11), is an assistant professor at Vanderbilt University School of Nursing, Nashville, Tennessee.

Sarah C. Craig, MS, RN (Introduction), is director of home care programs, Upjohn Healthcare Services, Kalamazoo, Michigan, and a director of the American Association for Continuity of Care.

John Feather, PhD (Chapter 12) is associate director, Western New York Geriatric Education Center, and research assistant professor, Department of Medicine, State University of New York at Buffalo, Buffalo, New York.

Evelyn G. Hartigan, EdD, RN, CNAA (coeditor; chapters 2, 3, 4, 6, and 7), is associate administrator, patient care services, and associate dean, nursing services, at the University of Utah Health Sciences Center, Salt Lake City, Utah.

Garnett Jones, RN (Chapter 8), is a consultant in discharge planning in Louisville, Kentucky.

Jo Keblusek, MSW, ACSW (Chapter 9), is director of the social work department, Little Company of Mary Hospital, Evergreen Park, Illinois.

Morris D. Kerstein, MD (Chapter 13), is professor, department of surgery, Tulane University School of Medicine, New Orleans, Louisiana.

Maureen K. Maguire, MS, RN, CNNA (Chapter 13), is assistant administrator, patient care and education, Department of Nursing, Tulane Medical Center, New Orleans, Louisiana.

Evelyn McNamara, MSW, ACSW (Chapter 5), is program coordinator, Eldercare, Johnston R. Bowman Health Center for the Elderly, Rush-Presbyterian-St. Luke's Medical Center, Chicago, Illinois.

Brenda C. Nave, RN (Chapter 10), is director, discharge planning department, Georgia Baptist Medical Center, Atlanta, Georgia.

Linda O. Nichols, PhD (Chapter 12), is a researcher, Veterans Administration Medical Center, Memphis, Tennessee.

Part I
INTRODUCTION

chapter 1

introduction

Sarah C. Craig

The first edition of *Discharge Planning for Continuity of Care* was compiled by staff members of the Virginia Regional Medical Program, Inc., and Blue Cross and Blue Shield of Virginia in 1974 and published by the National League for Nursing in 1976. As an important resource over the years, it has been read and reread by countless discharge planning professionals, has provided background information for innumerable educational sessions, and has been cited in bibliographies and references for major articles and publications in the field.

By publishing this second edition, the National League for Nursing is once again making valuable information available to discharge planning and continuity of care professionals. During this time of rapid change in health care delivery, it is important to preserve the history, background, and principles contained in this volume to provide a framework for new discharge planners. Experienced discharge planners will also benefit from getting back to these basics at regular intervals.

Much has happened in the decade since *Discharge Planning for Continuity of Care* was first published. According to Clement Bezold, "In business terms, in-patient hospital care is now in the mature or declining phase of its product life cycle."[1] It is being replaced by various forms of ambulatory care and other alternative levels of care. Increasingly sophisticated methods of utilization review, a declining birth rate, therapeutic breakthroughs in the practice of medicine, improved personal health habits, and the changing expectations of the health consumer have helped bring about a significant decrease in the number of patients being admitted to hospitals and the average number of days they spend there.

In 1983, Medicare implemented a prospective payment system that pays hospitals a flat rate for the patient's episode of care based on his or her diagnosis related group (DRG) rather than the actual cost of services rendered or number of patient days stayed. Thus hospitals may benefit financially from early discharge of patients. The DRG program has drawn attention to discharge planners and hospital systems for discharge planning.

Prospective payment has also intensified concern about the appropriateness of discharge plans for individual patients. Professional review organizations (PROs), under contracts with the government's Health Care Financing Administration (HCFA), will be monitoring hospitals' admission and readmission practices, the quality of care delivered, and unusually long or costly hospital stays for Medicare patients. At the local level, this review system is expected to dissuade hospitals from the following abuses of the prospective payment system:

- Manipulating the number and type of patients they admit to gain the most profitable reimbursement

- Undertreating Medicare beneficiaries

- Discharging patients too soon

- Inappropriately certifying that unusually long or expensive hospital stays are medically necessary.[2]

Employers in the private sector, increasingly frustrated because a large portion of their bill may be subsidizing hospitals for financial losses from the public-sector patient, are instituting their own cost-containment measures. Preadmission screening, utilization review, and attention to discharge plans for hospitalized employees provide a system of checks and balances to help ensure that insurance dollars are spent wisely—and some 10 percent of a company's payroll may be devoted to medical insurance.[3]

In the past, discharge planners have identified administrative support as the key component for a successful discharge planning program. Today, as another result of DRGs and cost-containment initiatives, many hospital administrators are heeding the American Hospital Association's admonition (first given in 1974) that "the establishment and maintenance of a discharge planning program are dependent on the acceptance and continued support of the hospital board, administration, medical staff, and other health care professionals." Administrators are recognizing that unless discharge planning is a "centralized, coordinated, interdisciplinary process," appropriate patient-centered discharge planning may happen only on an ad hoc basis.[4]

Even with administrative support and a broad institutional approach, turf and overlapping roles in the discharge planning process continue to be problematic for discharge planners, administrators, and other hospital staff. There appears to be unanimous agreement that the discharge planning process requires multidisciplinary input and interdisciplinary collaboration. However, there is little agreement as to which health care discipline is best suited to the discharge planning coordinator role, where that person and department should be located (directly under administration, in social service, in nursing, in utilization review, etc.), and which model should be followed.

Health care professionals seem to be finding it productive to address such divisive issues in an open and professional manner. In an effort to improve the state of the art, the American Association for Continuity of Care, a national organization for health professionals involved in discharge planning and continuity of care, convened a turf task force at its 1984 annual meeting. This task force defined the problem as follows:

> Discharge planning or providing continuity of care is by definition a multidisciplinary endeavor. As health care disciplines interface within the health care institution, with each other and with patients through discharge planning, their competition, misunderstanding, lack of respect, differing values and orientations, and self-protection interfere with effective patient care. These phenomena represent the "turf problem." In order to improve patient care through discharge planning, the turf problem must be addressed and resolved over time in each health care institution.[5]

The first suggested strategy for change? Gain administration's support to establish an interdisciplinary task force. Such a task force can do much to encourage cooperation within the institution and with the outside agencies helping to provide continuity of care for patients.

Turf is not the only problem plaguing discharge planners in their attempts to define their roles. From the beginning, discharge planners have been viewed and have viewed themselves as patient advocates. In the early 1900s, for example, Bellevue Hospital in New York City established a position for a nurse whose entire time and care was given to "befriending those about to be discharged." She accomplished this by inquiring into their circumstances, finding out whether they had home or friends to return to, and, if necessary, securing admission for them into some "curative or consolatory refuge." Similarly, a social worker employed by Dr. Cabot at Boston's Massachusetts General Hospital devoted attention to the patient's home environment as well as interpreting the hospital to the patient.[6]

Today discharge planners must provide similar functions in an era of cost and time constraints. They are seen by their administrators as cost shavers who can cut days off patient stays, thus saving the hospital a great deal of money. "Discharge quicker and sicker" or "treat 'em and street 'em" are phrases that mock the growing emphasis on shortening lengths of stay.

With earlier discharge, responsibility for care and rehabilitation may quickly shift from the hospital to the patient and family, leaving them confused and resentful. Certainly, this faster pace makes counseling patients about future care alternatives more difficult, especially when time is short and the alternatives difficult to identify and evaluate.[7]

Alternative delivery sites and modes for aftercare are developing rapidly, spurred by strong economic incentives in the marketplace. These increasing numbers of external agencies have targeted discharge planners as significant referral sources. Agencies compete to supply patients about to be discharged with posthospital services and goods. Ethical, professional, and legal considerations of what constitutes appropriate patient counseling and referral practices are of serious concern to discharge planners. In addition, how does the discharge planner schedule the time to see all those who wish to sell the merits of these programs and still have time to deal with the increased caseload he or she may be experiencing as a result of DRGs? Hospital discharge planners also encounter other "outsiders," such as home care coordinators and insurance and health maintenance organization case managers, who seek access to patient information and discharge plans. Such interactions usually promote continuity of care and are seen as beneficial if carried out according to jointly established job descriptions and protocol.

In the final analysis, the expanding universe of discharge planners seems to be having a positive effect on their professional growth. Through interactions within and outside of their institutions, discharge planners are educating others and being educated themselves. The specialized knowledge and the ever-increasing amount of information needed to carry out discharge planning in a high-speed, high-tech, highly competitive environment leads some experts to predict that discharge planning will soon be considered as a profession in its own right rather than "a foster child of one of the traditional health professions."[8]

Discharge planners are finding that the time they have spent learning discharge planning skills and developing expertise in continuity of care is translating into job security and employment opportunities, not only in the hospital setting but in the HMO, the urgent care facility, the durable medical equipment company, and the home health care field. There is, after all, assessment and planning for transition wherever health care delivery takes place.

Because of their special vantage point, experienced discharge planners are often able to provide a unique perspective at a time of confusion, conflict, and change for the health care industry. They are particularly qualified to focus attention on patients' needs for continuity of care and to promote and enhance linkages that heighten the quality of professional practice.

Part II
THE BASICS OF
DISCHARGE PLANNING

chapter 2

definitions, goals, benefits, principles

The health worker and discharge planner want to know:

- What is discharge planning?

- Who is it for? Why is it necessary? Will it guarantee quality patient care?

- How does a patient-centered program get started?

- Who does it? When does it take place? Where does it occur?

- How can it be paid for? Is it cost effective?

- Who should help plan a hospital or nursing home discharge planning program? Where does the health provider fit in?

- What will the institution gain? What are the expected outcomes for the patient?

- Will the community benefit? What if there is no place for the patient to be discharged *to*?

WHAT ARE DISCHARGE PLANNING AND CONTINUITY OF CARE?

Discharge planning, which aims to ensure continuity of care, helps sick and well persons and their families find the best solutions to their health problems, at the right time, from the appropriate source, at the best price, and on a continuous basis for the required period of time. Care often begins in one institution and continues uninterrupted in another if patient and health care personnel plan cooperatively. Effective discharge planning recognizes the danger of shifting problem patients from one health care agency to another and meticulously coordinates the efforts of all agencies and personnel to avoid such catastrophic occurrences.

Establishing a discharge planning program begins with an operational definition of discharge planning unique to the patient care institution and situation. "Discharge planning," "continuity of care," "medical care," and "comprehensive health care" are not synonymous terms. The following definitions may prove helpful as you plan your program.

Discharge planning is:

- "That part of the continuity of care process which is designed to prepare the patient or client for the next phase of care and to assist in making any necessary arrangements for that phase of care, whether it be self care, care by family members, or care by an organized health care provider."[1] The concept is simple: *organized planning* centered on the patient's health problems.

- A part of the overall plan of care for the patient that includes (1) assessing and identifying current and anticipated psychosocial and physiological needs; (2) planning appropriate continuing care to meet those needs when a change in or termination of services by the current health care provider occurs; and (3) preparing and referring the patient for admission to another organized health care service, or preparing the patient or client for self-care.[2]

- Working with the patient and family to arrange for appropriate health care services.

- In effect, a multidisciplinary team approach that ensures quality coordinated care. Discharge planning provides the mechanisms for providing continuous care, information about continuing health care requirements after discharge, appointments for follow-up medical supervision, and appropriate instructions for self-care.

Continuity of care is:

- A series of organized, connected patient-care events or activities that occur on a continuum even though the patient's need or desire for care varies, and even when health care is given by numerous providers.

- An ideal that requires (1) that the health care structure or system provide for and identify linkages among the health care providers; (2) that each provider within the system be identified as a contributor to a general health care plan for the individual; and (3) that there be planning, coordinating, communicating, referral, and follow-up to achieve the mutually agreed upon goals.[3]

Comprehensive personal health care is health care services for patients and families that includes four essential components: (1) health education, (2) personal preventive services, (3) diagnostic and therapeutic services, and (4) rehabilitative and restorative services.[4] A *health facility* is an organization designed, financed, equipped, staffed, and operated as an integral part of a comprehensive health care system. Discharge planning unites the various types of health facilities to ensure a continual flow of services to the patient.[5]

WHY IS DISCHARGE PLANNING A PATIENT'S RIGHT?

Individuals and families must be ensured appropriate entry points into an uninterrupted flow of health services. This is essential in ensuring that optimum levels of good health are maintained for the nation as a whole.

Twentieth-century medical knowledge has given providers the ability to cure many diseases and to control others. Therefore, quality medical and related personal health services have changed from a luxury to a necessity in today's society.[6] Americans regard good health and quality health care as the right of every individual. On November 17, 1972, the American Hospital Association included the following as one of the twelve items in its "Patient's Bill of Rights":

> The patient has the right to expect reasonable continuity of care. He has the right to know in advance what appointment times and physicians are available and where. The patient has the right to expect that the hospital will provide a mechanism whereby he is informed by his physician or a delegate of the physician of the patients' continuing health care requirements following discharge.[7]

WHAT ARE SOME GOALS OF DISCHARGE PLANNING?

Everyone involved in the discharge planning process will realize benefits if the following patient-centered goals are achieved:

- The patient and family actively participate in the discharge planning process.
- High-risk patients, or patients with potential discharge planning problems, are identified as soon as possible after admission to the facility.
- Solid collaborative and communication processes exist between and among all personnel involved in discharge planning.
- The most economical and appropriate options are selected.
- Current knowledge of available health care providers, programs, and resources is maintained.

WHAT ARE SOME ANTICIPATED REWARDS FOR THE PATIENT, PROVIDERS, AND COMMUNITY WHEN SOUND MANAGEMENT IS APPLIED TO DISCHARGE PLANNING PROGRAMS?

See Figure 2.1 for a model of a patient-centered discharge planning program.

- Overall responsibility for organized discharge planning is established, thus meeting the requirements of regulatory and accrediting bodies.
- The patient and family continue to be meaningfully involved in the discharge planning process, thus assuming their appropriate share of responsibility.
- There is effective utilization of personnel and facilities.
- There is appropriate use of community resources.
- Anticipatory planning and documentation should decrease the number of retroactive denials from insurance carriers and help hospitals provide effective care within diagnosis related group (DRG) cost constraints.
- There is appropriate utilization of health care services.
- There is an anticipated decrease in the number of relapses, hospital readmissions, and unnecessary emergency visits to hospitals.
- There is an improvement in public relations when institutions demonstrate responsiveness to patients' postdischarge needs.[8]
- The patient and family understand the need for aftercare and the cost of treatment.

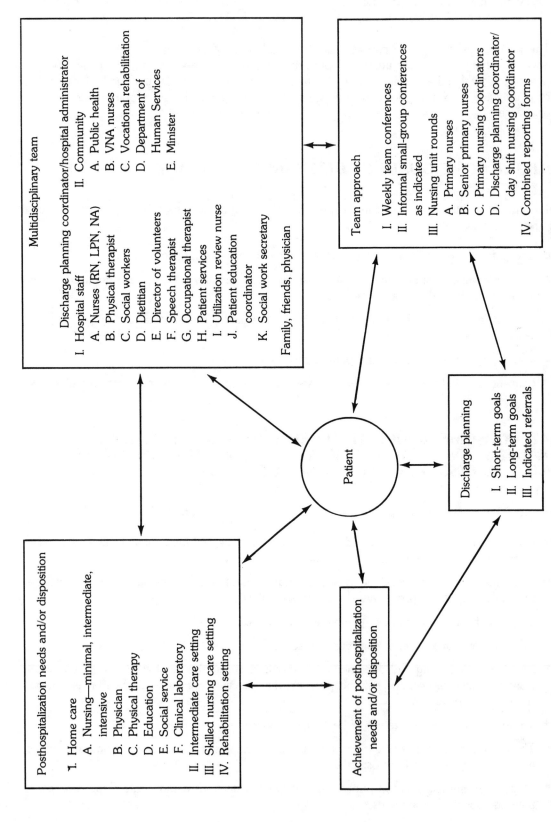

Figure 2.1. Johnson City Medical Center discharge planning model. (Source: Johnson City Medical Center, "Discharge Planning Model," *Discharge Planning Update*, Fall 1982, p. 33.)

- The discharge plan reduces the financial burden on the patient, family, facility, and third-party payer and meets the requirements of regulatory and accrediting bodies.

- Interdisciplinary and interagency planning and communication ensure the optimal utilization of appropriate resources and services.

- Documentation of the discharge planning process and systematic data collection provide adequate evidence for program continuity and quality assurance studies that enhance patient care.

- Community resources are mobilized to meet specific patient needs.

- Trauma and anxiety generated by movement from one level of care to another is minimized.

- Independent service units can blend care activities so that the system helps prolong the life for each component.

- Better utilization of health manpower will occur.

THE DISCHARGE PLANNING PROCESS: BASIC PRINCIPLES AND ELEMENTS

The planning process, which is applicable to individual patients or groups of patients within any given care setting, should begin when *a person enters the health delivery system*, especially those with chronic or complex problems requiring the assistance of multiple resources.

The discharge planner should use problem-solving techniques to:

- Diagnose and assess discharge planning needs.

- Identify major problems.

- Design a plan and set goals for the patient or the facility's program.

- Decide on and test action plans.

- Measure results.

- Evaluate the total program and make changes as needed.

The following are tasks that discharge planners must carry out:

- Select patient population groups that require discharge planning in order of priority; develop and use predetermined criteria to set priorities (for example, of 100 new admissions, decide who has the most urgent need for an immediate discharge plan).

- Develop administrative recognition and support, have specific staff members assigned to discharge planning, develop documentation and evaluation systems.

- Bring resources and the patient and family together.

- Inform the patient and family of the options available.

- Involve the patient and family in the planning process.

- Ensure a continuous flow of resources, information, and patient care data between a variety of care settings through formal and informal agreements with health care institutions, community agencies, and physicians' offices.

- Include multidisciplinary planning on a communitywide basis (for example, groups of discharge planners may hold periodic meetings to share ideas, solve problems, develop referral forms, etc.).

- Use a team approach that is integrated and coordinated and under the leadership of the discharge planning coordinator.

- Focus on identifying current patient problems and set up a mechanism for joint exploration of further problems.

- Consider the patient's previous care as it relates to the immediate need.

- Include patient education.

- Integrate and coordinate discharge planning activities with quality assurance programs within the institution.

- Provide a structured means of helping the physician plan for continuity of medical care (before, during, and after hospitalization).

- Include staff development programs on the subject of continuity of care.

- Identify community resources that are needed but unavailable.

- Develop written policies and procedures approved by appropriate administrative personnel.

- Define responsibilities for the discharge planning unit and agency personnel.

In summary, discharge planning is a health care management process necessary to identify and resolve simple and complex patient health problems. The primary beneficiary of this systematic approach to the delivery of care should be the patient. The various components of the delivery system should improve their productivity by centering attention on patient needs.

The success of a discharge planning program depends upon appraising need and matching that need as closely as possible with available resources. Discharge planning is dependent upon the following six variables:

1. Degree of illness or health

2. Expected outcome of care

3. Duration or length of care needed

4. Types of services required

5. Addition of complications

6. Resources available

Continuity of patient care must be planned for. Every patient should have the opportunity to reach his maximum potential for recovery. Planning for continuity of care includes planning for the transfer of patients between units within a hospital or nursing home, planning for discharge of a patient from the hospital to the home or to another care facility, and planning for use of resources within the community that supplement and reinforce the discharge planning activities of the health care facilities.

Institutions and personnel responsible for patient care are in a position to establish coordinated and systematic admissions and discharge processes that will resolve patient problems. The alternative to systematic patient care is a series of professional activities that are disjointed, not patient centered, and costly and that may often leave patient needs unmet.

chapter 3

finance and regulations

The discharge planner needs to understand:

- How the Medicare prospective payment system influences planned admissions, discharge planning, and earlier discharges.

- Which diagnosis related groups (DRGs) significantly affect the individual hospital.

- The financial implications of transferring patients to facilities that are, or are not, exempt from prospective pricing regulations.

- How quality assurance programs, utilization review, and discharge planning are interconnected.

HOW DOES THE CHANGING HEALTH SYSTEM AFFECT ADMISSION AND DISCHARGE PRACTICES?

Consumer groups, the federal government, third-party payers, and health professionals are concerned about quality assurance, cost control, and efficiency. One provider alone or the single health professional can no longer fulfill all the patient's need for health services.

The Tax Equity and Fiscal Responsibility Act of 1982 (Public Law 97-248) and the enactment of Section 223, the prospective payment system for Medicare (effective with the fiscal year that began on October 1, 1983), signaled many changes in health care philosophy. "Current thinking is that if hospitals are paid a flat illness-specific amount that is set prospectively—before services are rendered—and that is independent of a patient's length of stay and services received, they would function more effectively. In other words, prospective flat amounts would encourage hospitals to weigh each service's contribution to a patient's well-being carefully and to avoid unnecessary stays and ancillary services because 'excess care' would automatically reduce net revenue."[1] By establishing financial incentives for institutions to keep their costs below Medicare's preset prices, the government hopes to encourage cost-conscious management and cost-effective utilization of clinical services.

"Improving hospital financial performance under prospective payment will require a combination of strategies to reduce Medicare costs and manage total revenues . . . strategies that will yield the greatest benefit to the hospital will concentrate on managing cost by . . . intensive discharge planning and the use of referral arrangements with community agencies and other providers."[2] The discharge planner who responsibly coordinates input from other health professionals with an appropriate assessment of the patient's and family's needs, problems, and available resources is in a unique position to provide an effective plan for continuity of care. The advent of prospective payment utilizing DRGs, combined with the growth in the Medicare population, have made effective discharge planning essential for both quality patient care and the financial survival of the hospital.[3]

WEIGHTS OF VARIOUS DRGs

Just as extensive discharge planning is not appropriate for all patients, all DRGs are not of equal importance to the institution. According to the American Hospital Association, in 1980, 100 of the 470 DRGs included approximately 80 percent of all Medicare discharges. In that year, 27 DRGs included 50 percent of all Medicare patients, and 8 DRGs included 25 percent of all Medicare patients.

Within each Major Diagnostic Category (MDC), three or four DRGs typically account for the majority of patients classified into that MDC. For example, in MDC 05, Diseases and Disorders of the Circulatory System, more than 50 percent of all patients are classified into four DRGs and 75 percent of all patients are classified into eight DRGs. In MDC 01, Diseases and Disorders of the Nervous System, 50 percent of all patients are classified into two DRGs, while six DRGs account for 75 percent of all admissions. In general, a few DRGs are extremely important, whereas many DRGs are rarely used, due to the characteristics of the hospital's Medicare patients.[4]

The discharge planner should determine which DRGs account for the majority of Medicare patients within the institution. Although this information may have no immediate importance, it may prove valuable when she attempts to prioritize cases, requests additional assistance, or communicates with other health professionals, especially administration and financial officers.

TRANSFER TO EXEMPT OR NONEXEMPT UNITS OR INSTITUTIONS

Discharge planning should be carried out in keeping with varying community resources and with due regard for prospective pricing. The full DRG price, including any outlier payments, is paid automatically only to the hospital that discharges the patient to his home or to an exempt provider, such as a skilled nursing facility, a long term care hospital, a children's hospital, a psychiatric hospital, or a rehabilitation hospital. Special provisions for prospective payment apply to hospitals that meet the criteria established for regional referral centers, disproportionate-share hospitals, cancer hospitals, and sole community providers.[5]

Reimbursement to both the receiving and transferring institutions is affected by their exempt or nonexempt status. Administrative policies should be developed that specify how choices should be made among alternatives; the impact of such transfers on the institution's fiscal policies; and what financial responsibilities the patient and family might be expected to assume.

WHAT DO REGULATORY AGENCIES SAY ABOUT DISCHARGE PLANNING?

Discharge planning is mandated by many accrediting, licensing, and professional organizations. In the *Accreditation Manual for Hospitals*, published by the Joint Commission on Accreditation of Hospitals (JCAH), repeated reference is made to discharge planning and continuity of care. For instance, Nursing Services Standard IV states, "The [nursing care] plan shall include nursing measures that will facilitate the medical care prescribed and that will restore, maintain, or promote the patient's well-being. As appropriate, such measures should include physiological, psychosocial, and environmental factors; patient/family education; and patient discharge planning."[6]

Utilization Review Standard 1, lines 25–35 of the JCAH *Manual* states that "to facilitate discharge as soon as an acute level of care is no longer required, discharge planning shall be initiated as early as a determination of the need for such activity can be made. Criteria for initiating discharge planning may be developed to identify patients whose diagnoses, problems or psychosocial circumstances usually require discharge planning. The utilization review plan may specify the situation in which nonphysician health care professionals may initiate preparations for discharge planning. Discharge planning should not be limited to the placement in long term care facilities, but shall include provision for, or referral to, services that may be required to improve or maintain the patient's health status."[7]

The introduction to the American Hospital Association's *Guidelines for Discharge Planning* states that "coordinated discharge planning functions are essential for hospitals to maintain high-quality patient care. Discharge planning is important because it facilitates appropriate patient and family decision making. In addition, it can also help reduce length of stay and the rate of increase of health costs."[8]

The American Nurses' Association Division on Medical-Surgical Nursing Practice and the Division on Community Health Nursing Practice have issued a statement, *Continuity of Care and Discharge Planning Programs*. In this pamphlet rationales for discharge planning are identified, functions of discharge planning and referral are specified, and types of discharge planning programs are described. The conclusion of this policy statement declares that the "American Nurses' Association believes that the patient or client has a right to expect that his discharge from a health care provider is planned. Not every patient/client will need a referral to another institution, but every patient/client should be assessed for continuing needs."[9]

The following recommendations from the Professional Standards Review Organizations manual (superseded by the Professional Review Organizations) remain valid for today's discharge planner:

> Where problems in post-discharge care or discharge placement are anticipated, discharge planning should be initiated as soon as possible after admission to the facility. Discharge planning should include both preparation of the patient for the next level of care and arrangement for placement in the appropriate health care setting. Information needed for the discharge planning process includes:
>
> a) Prior health care status of the patient (i.e., was the patient managing his own care, receiving care in his home or in some type of extended care facility?)
>
> b) Current level of care required.
>
> c) Projected level(s) of care needed.
>
> d) Projected time frame for moving patient to next level of care.
>
> e) Therapy(ies) and teaching that must be accomplished prior to discharge.
>
> f) Resources available for post-hospital care; and
>
> g) Mechanisms for facilitating transfer to other levels of care.[10]

PRESSURE FROM MEDICARE-MEDICAID UTILIZATION REVIEW COMMITTEE

At a certain time in the patient's treatment, the patient and his physician are notified of the utilization review committee's decision about his recommended discharge date. At the same time, the committee may advise the patient's prepayment or insurance carrier that benefits beyond the recommended discharge date are not medically necessary. The discharge planning program acts to assist the patient and physician with movement to home or another facility. This does not mean that the patient must leave the nursing home or hospital. It may mean that he will personally pay some or all charges for services provided past the recommended discharge date. Effective, timely discharge planning may save the patient and family this additional expense.

chapter 4

the service population

> **The discharge planner should explore these questions:**
>
> ● Do all patients require admission and discharge planning?
>
> ● What specific types of patients need discharge planning?
>
> ● Which patients require discharge planning services?
>
> ● How can hospital patients be identified and priorities set?
>
> ● Why is home care preferable to institutional care for many patients?
>
> ● Do only Medicare patients require discharge planning?

DO ALL PATIENTS REQUIRE ADMISSION AND DISCHARGE PLANNING?

In reality *all* patients require some type of planning at the time of admission to a facility. The patient's status should be assessed and his needs anticipated, whether the plans made are simple or complex. For example, some patients require only the date of their next appointment with the primary physician or self-care instructions from the primary professional nurse. Other patients and families need detailed educational or other assistance that may involve many different health care professionals. Some patients require extensive assistance and planning to understand their needs and prepare for transfer to an extended care facility. In any case, the first step for the discharge planner is to evaluate the patient's needs:

> The key word in discharge planning is "evaluate"—evaluate for what? Evaluate for everything! This is a large order, but the comprehensive mind of the discharge planner catalogues statistical

information on the patient, such as:

—What is the patient's diagnosis?

—What medications are being taken by the patient?

—How are the medications being administered (p.o. IM, IV, NG—other)?

—What therapies are being used in the hospital—will they continue after the patient is discharged from the hospital?

—How old is the patient?

—Where does the patient live?

—Does the patient live alone?

—What type of income does the patient have—Social Security? Medicaid? Financially independent?

A breakdown of elements which identify needs for patients in terms of posthospital care are conceptually identified as follows:

—Types of Nursing Care:

—Syringe Feeding

—Sterile Dressing

—Prosthesis Care

—Special Skin Care

—Decubitus Care

—Catheterization

—Foley/Indwelling Catheter Care

—Suprapubic Catheter Care

—Oxygen

—Fracture Care

—Oral Suction

—Tracheostomy Care

—Gastrostomy Care

—Inhalation Therapy

—Irrigations

—Enemas

—Colostomy Care

—Ileostomy Care

—Other

Rehabilitation Service Care:

—Physical Therapy

—Speech Therapy

—Occupational Therapy

—Bowel and Bladder Training

—Prosthesis Training

—Other

Functioning Identification:

—Speech Problem

—Blindness

—Fecal Incontinence

—Aphasia

—Urinary Incontinence

—Bedfast

—Deafness

—Other

Do these elements require total or partial care?

—Mental Status of the Patient:

—Alert

—Disoriented

—Forgetful

—Comatose

—Semicomatose

—Controlled with Medication

—Other

Behavior Problems the Patient Displays:

—Confusion

—Hyperactivity

—Disruptive

—Withdrawn

—Other[1]

WHAT SPECIFIC TYPES OF PATIENTS NEED DISCHARGE PLANNING?

It is advisable to identify the types of patients in each institution that have the most intense needs for discharge planning. These needs may arise from the disease process itself, the types of surgical intervention, the patient's inability to manage self-care, inappropriate home environment, economic difficulties, or the absence of caring relatives or friends.

A pragmatic approach is to determine what patients usually require discharge planning services. This information is then used as a data base for the development of a computer program that will automatically identify (and alert the discharge planner to) those patients and families who are likely to require assistance.

The primary care nurse and the head nurse on each nursing unit are in ideal positions to identify the "nonroutine" patients who should be referred to the discharge planning staff. The primary care nurse should be able to identify the patient with unique postdischarge needs. (For example: the newly invalid mother who is solely responsible for a retarded child.) The head nurse will be knowledgeable about newly instituted procedures or treatments that may necessitate prolonged home care. It is crucial that nursing service personnel not only seek and appropriately document such information but also effectively communicate it in a timely manner to administrative and discharge planning personnel.

WHICH PATIENTS REQUIRE DISCHARGE PLANNING SERVICES?

There is no single, universally applicable formula for determining which patients will benefit most from discharge planning assistance. The types of patients served and the services they require will vary from institution to institution with geographic location and the socioeconomic status of the service population. The following list (developed by the University Hospital, University of Utah Medical Center, Salt Lake City, Utah) is provided as an example of one institution's guidelines:

The presence of any one of the following criteria present upon admission (or which develops subsequently) triggers automatic social work–nursing intervention and initiation of early discharge planning:

1. Any person age 70 or older who is living alone.

2. Any person age 70 or over admitted to the hospital for total joint replacement.

3. Any person admitted to the hospital who does not reside in the area normally served by the University Hospital in Salt Lake City.

4. Patients who have attempted suicide in the past two years, or who are considered high suicide risks.

5. Patients of all ages who are admitted from or anticipate being transferred to nursing homes, residential care homes, or specialty hospitals.

6. Patients in need of supportive follow-up treatment, teaching, and/or referral to appropriate community agencies.

7. Patients who are known to be followed by community agencies at the time of admission and who may require continued follow-up after discharge.

8. Patients who have been hospitalized three or more times during the preceding year.

9. Patients with inadequate financial resources.

10. Patients with congenital abnormalities that impair or impede normal growth and body function.

11. Patients suffering from multiple trauma.

12. Patients with progressive neurological, neuromuscular, metabolic, cerebrovascular, or renal disease with resulting impairment.

13. All psychiatric patients.

14. Patients who show evidence of physical or emotional abuse upon admission to the hospital.

15. All severely visually impaired patients.[2]

HOW CAN HOSPITAL PATIENTS BE IDENTIFIED AND PRIORITIES SET?

The Neonate

Newborns with life-threatening congenital abnormalities are usually transferred immediately to perinatal centers or a neonatal ICU. The discharge planner should be informed of such interagency or interhospital moves. However, it is the infant with less severe problems who may provide the greatest challenge for the discharge planner. The neonate with an abnormal birth weight, a single parent, a teenage mother, or whose parents are impoverished or substance abusers may require intensive services or referral to the public health nurse.

The discharge planner may be alerted to these problems by the delivery room or nursery nurse or may do independent case finding, using information obtained from admission forms or the mother's prenatal record or admission history. The primary nurse's assessment of inappropriate or inadequate maternal–child bonding may indicate the need for postdischarge assistance. Most health departments have referral priority lists that the discharge planner should be aware of.

Pediatric Patients

The desirability of avoiding the admission of pediatric patients to the hospital except in cases of very acute, episodic illness is well known. Coordinated home care service can and should be used in all suitable cases either to prevent admission or shorten length of stay.

The family of any child admitted with a frightening diagnosis or for unusual surgical intervention usually requires specialized aid when the child leaves the hospital. Discharge planning for the child starts with helping him understand and accept the illness, physician, and hospital system. Often a child's behavior that is interpreted as "good" is actually "scared" behavior. The child is quiet because he doesn't know what is going to happen to him. Here is an excellent opportunity for discharge planning and education; the parents should be involved in the process as well as the child.

Maternity Patients and Young Mothers

The complications of pregnancy and selected normal deliveries are generally considered appropriate conditions for pre- and posthospital home care evaluation. Medically coordinated home care for many prenatal and postpartum patients is desirable therapeutically and financially. The average length of stay for routine deliveries in the Middle Atlantic States in 1961 was 5.3 days.[3] By 1983, the average length of stay nationwide for an uncomplicated vaginal delivery was 2.8 days.[4] By 1984, some hospitals were discharging these patients 8 hours after delivery.

Earlier hospital discharge for properly evaluated maternity patients is advantageous because it:

- Reduces the risk of hospital-borne infections.

- Allows for the adequate preparation of the mother and family members to care for their newborn at home.

- Provides an opportunity for the social worker, public health nurse, or other health worker to recognize and aid in the solution of family health problems.

- Permits savings resulting from earlier hospital discharges to be used for lower cost coordinated home care services.[5]

Surgical Patients and Patients with Acute Illness

Doctors, nurses, and social workers can aid in discharge planning when they are aware of how much surgery can disrupt a person's life. Often patients who have unresolved problems request an additional stay in the hospital. If admission and discharge planning have been adequate, the patient is more willing to accept the physician's and other professionals' recommendations.

Adult Patients Suffering From Multiple Chronic Illness

This group patients with multiple medical diagnoses who, after a period of hospitalization, still require a prolonged convalescence and further intermittent medical and nursing care, but not hospitalization. These patients include those suffering from heart disease (more than half of this group), cancer and rheumatoid arthritis (20 percent), and convalescing hip fractures (5 percent). The remaining 25 percent are patients with long-term illnesses such as emphysema, diabetes, asthma, Parkinson's disease, diverticulitis, multiple sclerosis, and cardiovascular accidents.

Planning for the health care of these patients in the community is difficult, but they can be assisted to a varying extent by discharging them to home care, long term care facilities, or day care centers, if the resources are available.

Geriatric Patients

In discussing the needs of the aging, it is necessary to consider both their medical and nonmedical needs after discharge from a facility. A geriatric patient needs specialized care.

Only a small percent of elderly individuals (those 65 years of age and older) need assistance to carry out activities of daily living. The real problems relating to discharge and placement of older patients involve those without homes or relatives capable of caring for them or helping them to care for themselves.

When such a patient is discharged from the hospital, alternatives must be found for his care. These include skilled nursing facilities, custodial care facilities, foster homes, day care, and his own home where a home care program has been designed for him. The families of aging preterminal or terminal patients are often too emotionally involved to make the necessary plans for care outside the hospital or nursing home.

Emotionally Labile or Disturbed Patients

Current philosophy in the treatment of mental illness dictates that, insofar as possible, treatment should be provided within the community. The emotionally labile or disturbed patient has difficulty adjusting to problems of convalescence. The discharge needs of the mentally ill patient who has been hospitalized in his own community (e.g., in the local general hospital) are much the same as those of the medical or surgical patient in that same environment. The imposition of treatment regimens in hospitals, away from the patient's usual surroundings, accentuates the mentally ill patient's already extensive feelings of personal alienation and concurrently supports society's image of the mentally ill as dependent. Discharge planning for these patients may include outpatient treatment or continued medication and other services. Additionally, it may include:

- A provision for halfway-house services, or nursing home care for the patient who is not prepared to return directly to independent living.

- Establishing food service and resocialization programs for the patient who is able to maintain himself independently or live with his family.

- Rehabilitative services to train the patient for employment.

- Combinations of the basic services listed above.

Patients Who Have Had Radical or Mutilating Surgery

This group includes those patients whose surgery results in a markedly changed life-style as well as environmental shifts and changes in family relationships:

- Removal of kidney, requiring home or outpatient dialysis (dialysis assistance for life).
- Changed body functioning, such as ostomy surgery.
- Radical neck or face reconstruction.
- Bilateral arm or leg amputation.
- Intrapsychic adjustments.
- Cardiovascular reconstruction.

If these patients must be discharged to another institution for long term or preterminal or hospice care, this may represent as much of a crisis as admission. Special crisis intervention by health care personnel may be required. Because of the fears and anxieties of the patient and family, the discharge planner should assess the patient's ability to adjust to the many ramifications of his illness.

Patients included in this radical surgery group generally have special posthospital convalescent nursing problems. Also included in this group are debilitated patients who must return to heavy home responsibilities (such as children, aging parents, chronically ill mates, and the like).

Emergency Department Patients

The total patient care provided for emergency department patients should include discharge planning. Because of the unexpected nature of the illness or injury, the emergency patient may not have either an acceptance or understanding of his condition.

Emergency patients are, in general, overlooked by discharge planners. There are really two types of discharge from an emergency department: discharge into the hospital and discharge into the community. For patients who are admitted to the hospital, the emergency department social worker may make a brief social assessment and refer the patient to the inpatient social worker or discharge planner.

The more difficult discharge task in the emergency department, however, is discharge to the community. Although discharge planning is always somewhat different for each patient, there are usually six questions that need be asked. These questions summarize the goal of discharge planning in the emergency department, which is to protect the patient and others from the further harm that might be caused by premature or unassisted discharge.

The questions that should be asked about every emergency patient who is to be discharged to the community are:

- Is the patient ready for discharge?
- Has the patient received all the medical services he needs right now?
- Does the patient have a safe and adequate place to go?
- Does the patient have understandable, available, and agreed-upon follow-up arrangements?
- What risks point to need for immediate social work intervention?
- Is discharging this patient likely to cause harm to the patient or others?[6]

Patients without Families and Patients in the Poverty Groups

Usually patients in these groups are dependent on large bureaucratic community agencies. Their problems may be more those of displacement than of placement. Often their problems are temporarily "solved" by referring them to facilities willing to offer a bed rather than to the institution that can best meet their needs. In a survey of several Pennsylvania hospitals, it was found that a large percentage of patients in each institution could be discharged if supportive care were offered (e.g., community housing). This is in order that:

● No person will be confined to an institution unless absolutely necessary.

● Every attempt will be made to retain the patient in his own home.

● In the absence of a home, a foster home or some type of community living will be secured that will permit him to remain with friends.

Foster home placement is the ideal solution for patients who lack a home and need familylike supportive care. Since foster homes are scarce, an alternative is public housing that offers services similar to a foster home at a cost that is not prohibitive to the patient.[7]

WHY IS HOME CARE PREFERABLE TO INSTITUTIONAL CARE FOR MANY PATIENTS?

Coordinated home care prevents the development of the passive-dependent state engendered by long hospitalization. Patients in extended care facilities often lose their initiative and regress almost to a vegetative state. Patients tend to keep up their desire to care for themselves at home.

Long-term illness frequently brings on depression and despair. The social service and psychiatric assistance components of a home care program help counteract this despondency and assist in emotional adjustment. The patient generally seems happier in his own home. In addition, the patient is not exposed to the illnesses of other patients or to the picture of suffering and death he might see in an institution. These experiences frequently aggravate patients' depression and despair.

The cost of coordinated home care is approximately one-fourth the cost of inpatient hospital care. This is extremely important to patients who have no hospitalization insurance or who have exhausted their insurance.

At home, the patient retains his identity and sense of usefulness. He can look after his home or business in an advisory or supervisory capacity. An organized home care program should have resources, services and personnel to facilitate this for the patient and his family. Often, this is crucial in the ability of a family to cope with a long illness.

TO WHOM CAN YOUR FACILITY PROVIDE DISCHARGE SERVICES? DO ONLY MEDICARE PATIENTS REQUIRE DISCHARGE PLANNING?

Medicare clearly outlines in operational and policy manuals what should be happening to a patient admitted to a home care program, a skilled nursing facility, or a hospital to ensure maximum reimbursement. Likewise the total health care system, regardless of payment source, also attempts to establish definitions and criteria that will enable personnel to understand who should be in the different levels of care. In addition to these general guidelines, it may be helpful to consider the following:

● The Utilization Review Committee may determine the need for discharge planning to satisfy some financing program.

● The availability of qualified personnel may determine the number and type of patients per month who will receive discharge assistance. For example, some hospitals and nursing homes have no designated discharge planner.

● The facility's administrative policy and budgetary support may be determining factors.

- The patient population mix and service needs will influence which patient groups will receive discharge service. For example, some hospitals have an extremely high Medicare and Medicaid admission rate; some nursing homes are licensed primarily for the intermediate level of care.

Financing sources should not completely dominate the decision to provide discharge planning service. Hospitals have a responsibility to assist patients with medical and related nonmedical problems. "Any patient who packs his suitcase for the hospital includes more than a toothbrush, a pair of pajamas and a bathrobe—he adds his worries, his concerns, his anxieties, and his fears, which involve him and his family as well as his community."[8]

The success of any hospital discharge planning program depends on how well the community understands and can provide for the posthospital needs of the patient. Success also depends on how well the hospital discharge planning personnel utilize existing community resources to successfully spot all patients with after-care needs.

patient and family involvement

Evelyn McNamara

The discharge planner should ask:

- For whom am I planning?

- Do I really know who these people are?

- Did I really hear what they said?

- Do I understand what they want and why?

- What can the patient and family really manage?

FOR WHOM IS DISCHARGE PLANNING? CONSIDER THE PATIENT AND FAMILY

Developing a discharge planning program includes defining the types of patients and problems for whom planning will be provided. Age categories, physical disabilities, certain diagnoses and treatments, repeated hospital admissions, and demographic and socioeconomic factors were listed in Chapter 4 as criteria for selecting patients. It is essential to discharge planning to learn to recognize the individuality of the people for whom the discharge planning program is created and what influence they will have on the process and the outcomes.

The American Hospital Association's *Introduction to Discharge Planning* defines "successful discharge planning" as a "centralized coordinated interdisciplinary process that ensures that all patients have a plan for continuing care after they leave the hospital. The plan should reflect both the patient's and the families' internal and external social, emotional, medical and psychological needs and assets."[1] Appropriate involvement of the patient and significant others may be the single most important part of an organized discharge plan.

Here the term *family* can mean persons related to the patient by blood, marriage, friendship, neighborhood, or guardianship. To involve the patient and family in the discharge planning process will mean gaining up-to-date knowledge of the individual and his particular situation. Important in that sentence are the words *planning process*, rather than just involvement in "the plan." Patients and their families have life histories, relationships, values, assets, and attitudes. They have rights and responsibilities that must be part of planning for their continuity of care and continuity of living. Patients and families must be informed of the options open to them and of the dangers of certain choices. They must be recognized as individuals whose life-styles, self-images, relationships, social and emotional functioning, and physical condition may and probably will be changed by the patient's illness, treatment, and prognosis.

Much is said today about the patient's autonomy and decision making in opposition to the paternalism of the medical system. Illness and treatment do alter a person's autonomy, but this does not grant to the medical care system the control and total responsibility for planning. The patient and family have a right to make decisions and a responsibility to know what goes into making a decision. They also have the right to choose an answer that meets their needs and provides for their good rather than what is perceived to be best by others. They even have the right to choose what does not appear to be for their good.

The decisions to be made are often momentous, as they involve changes that may have a major effect on a number of lives. Decision making may be the most important role carried out by the patient and family. The planner's responsibility is to provide the information, counseling, and support needed to make that decision.

Early involvement of the patient and related others and clarification of their role and responsibility to carry out that role is essential. Involve all in the goal setting as well as the plan itself. Obtaining this participation is sometimes difficult. Participation depends on the decision maker's social support network, belief that he can choose, and how much he feels compelled to comply with the wishes or demands of physician or family. Finally, hope may be a factor.[2]

Also, families and significant others have the right and responsibility *along with the patient* to become involved early in planning for after care; to be informed of alternatives, resources, risks, patient attitudes and preferences; to be listened to and heard; to seek other sources of counseling and planning; to accept wholly or only partially the plan in which they have participated; and to reject *your* plan. This rejection will carry with it a large responsibility for living with the risks involved, the drains and strains on resources and relationships. With a patient who is competent (and this is a hard word to define) these rights and responsibilities should be seen as shared.

WHO ARE THE PATIENT AND FAMILY?

To accord these rights and enable the patient and family to assume their responsibilities, the discharge planner and others involved in care need to know who this patient was and is. Ask these questions. Learn the answers. Remember that patients are not just the aged, or the poor, or the chronically ill or physically limited.

- Where did he come from? How long has he lived like that? Maybe he is 85 and has lived for five years in an apartment up three flights of stairs with four cats.

- What was she doing before the hospitalization? Was she the cook at the local diner?

- Who is really related to or involved with her? An elderly gentleman comes every day and says he is her next-door neighbor and only helper. Or she has three sons but a niece is the one who comes daily.

- What is the patient's life-style? daily patterns? The mother works and the children eat at will and mostly junk food. The child is now diagnosed as diabetic.

- Is physical activity or freedom from responsibility of major importance?

- What is the patient's ethnic or cultural background? The German-born wife says, "But in our country you never let your husband be cared for by someone else or in another place."

Can you learn enough about the patient to know:

- How he handled stress, problems, success or failure, or anger? Perhaps he is always outwardly calm, not verbally expressive. Will this mean you will not know his true reactions?

- Who appears to be the decision maker or the greatest influence?

- What strengths can you identify that will help in planning?

- Has he always defied the system?

- Can the patient and family communicate? Do they?

- How did they cope with previous illnesses and plans?

These answers, plus the information usually obtained in an admission history (or the nurse or social worker's review) on finances, physical environment, marital status, mental status, and health care patterns will give you a better picture of the person with whom you are planning.

Next look at the patient and others in relation to this illness (diagnoses, treatments, prognosis), the information they have and will receive about the future, the recommendations for establishing continuity of care:

- What were the patient or family told?

- What do you believe they heard?

- Have changes in mobility, speech, self-care, or cognition been accepted by patient and by others?

- What could these changes mean in terms of relationships and altered responsibility? (The patient has always paid the bills, repaired the house, driven the car, and written the letters. Now he has had a stroke.)

- Can the family handle the necessary changes?

- How does the dependency that remains affect the care to be given? (The patient has always been proud of her ability to care for herself and has never let anyone help her bathe or dress.)

- Do you see different interactions since planning began?

- Has the family withdrawn? Has the patient pushed others away? Why? How?

- What are the patient's and family's feelings about death and disability?

As planning goes forward you will need to find out more about who the patient and family really are and what help they will actually need, want, accept, and utilize. Clearly the planning will include specific arrangements for ongoing medical care; referrals for social and financial assistance; and identification of resources such as home care, equipment, nursing home, sheltered living, adapted house, caretakers.

Knowing the patient and family and helping them to take on the responsibility for not only the decision but the ongoing plan may require more knowledge and understanding, such as:

- Can the patient and family manage to carry out the plan after the hospital supports are gone?

- What are their attitudes toward "outside help"?

- Is there an alternative in the patient's plan?

- Do the patient and family know and accept the changes and risks involved? Do you?

- Is this to be a long-term or an interim plan?

- Is institutional care totally unacceptable?

- What does return home of a disabled or dependent person do to relationships? to the environment? to life-styles?

- What are the positive aspects of the particular plan?

- Can you, the planner, carry through with a plan that is culturally, socially, physically different than what you believe is appropriate?

- What do you do when there is conflict between patient and caretakers about what is the "best" or "right" plan?

- How much autonomy are the discharge planner, physician, and others willing to give?

Now, go back and ask again:

- For whom are we planning?

- Do we know really who these people are?

- Have we really heard what they are saying and do we understand what they are doing, what they want, and what they can manage?

From all these questions and answers one can begin to know who the patient is, what can be expected from him, what he has to do, and why. To obtain and use all this knowledge may seem impossible. It may take time that is seemingly unavailable.

The pressures of DRGs, third-party payer reviews, and staff shortages all call for plans that are enacted expeditiously. Consider, however, the plans that cannot be executed or that fall apart, the readmissions that might have been avoided or delayed if the planning had been individualized.

Many of the questions raised here can be answered by primary caregivers through their daily involvement and relationship with the patient. Physicians, therapists, clinical specialists, social worker, volunteers—all of whom observe and interact with the patient and family—can provide some of the answers. The patient and related others will give you much of the information you need as you carefully listen and observe. Include the patient in patient care conferences whenever possible; include the family from the beginning. Plan *with*, not *for*; remember that it is not your plan but that of the patient and family.

PROBLEMS FOR THE DISCHARGE PLANNER

"Discharge planning for continuity of care" at times may seem to be a self-contradictory phrase: the choices available for posthospital care may be limited and the decisions made by patient and family risky and ill-considered.

The problem for the discharge planner is often to examine what is right and what is good. Sometimes what is most needed is not available, and what the health care workers want is not possible or acceptable to patient and family.

Writing of ethical issues facing discharge planners, Thomas Holland says that "practitioners are expected to be supportive, insightful, protective, helpful, and controlling when necessary and highly ethical in all their judgements and actions." He adds, "They are to use their influence over people's lives in constructive ways—yet what does it mean to be helpful and constructive in problem situations . . . ?"[3]

At the beginning of this chapter it was stressed that the discharge planner must consider a range of attitudes, values, behaviors, relationships, problems, and strengths as essential to the provision of a discharge plan relevant to the patient, to the medical problem, and to the constraints of the institution and the present payment sources. How does one consider all these influences and needs and remain "supportive, . . . helpful, and controlling" in such instances as the following:

Mrs. Brown has had a massive CVA resulting in total right-sided paralysis, speech impairment, and apparent memory loss. All professionals involved recommend transfer to either a nursing home or a rehabilitation facility. Her husband (68 years old) and a single daughter (28 years old) are her only family. They wish to take Mrs. Brown home to care for her and insist that they need no formal instruction in her care. Mrs. Brown is 58, her insurance does not cover home health nursing, and the family budget will provide no more than $75 per week for additional assistance.

Mrs. Jones is a 37-year-old mother of five children (ages 15, 13, 11, 9, and 2). She lives in a trilevel house. Cooking, laundry facilities, and the only bathroom are on separate floors. Mrs. Jones has a full-length cast on her right leg for healing a severe compound fracture of the tibia and fibula. Mr. Jones will be out of the country for an extended period of time. Mrs. Jones does not feel that she needs the services of a homemaker and refuses all offers to make arrangements for assistance.

Mrs. Brown returns home, as her family wishes. Do you feel that you did all you could to help husband and daughter understand (not just be told) the extent of care and the physical, emotional, and financial drains that will take place? Have they had time to realize Mrs. Brown's incapacity and apparent inability to participate in her home care? Or do they deny her dependence and expect that she will soon be functioning like her old self? While formal instruction in her care is refused, what instruction has been given informally and through example as she has been hospitalized? Have resources even within that $75 been uncovered or a volunteer support system been discussed? What does a nursing home mean to this family? Remember the rights of family and patient to make decisions, even risky ones. Mrs. Brown's family will probably take her home. Physicians will be concerned; may be even angry. The discharge planner will feel unsuccessful because of the risks and strains and possible failure of the plan. But one cannot take on the whole responsibility for the decision making; one must learn also that life-styles, including willingness to accept sacrifices and live with burdens, vary and that what is good to you may be the wrong thing for others. You cannot carry the whole burden of the plan and its consequences. Inform, communicate, listen, understand, and do not consider that there was no discharge planning.

When one looks at Mrs. Jones again one has to ask the questions about relationships and strengths and weaknesses of patient and family. Do you know how much the children already do in the daily management of that household? Do they cook, clean, do laundry? Maybe a clean house is not the prime concern. Is Mrs. Jones willing and are they to have a child bring her a bed pan or help her bathe if she chooses to live on a floor without a bathroom? Can they adapt meals to where she is? Have they already learned to cope without Mr. Jones for lengthy periods? Again, knowing the answers to some of these questions should help the discharge planner complete the actual discharge and offer sufficient guidance. Also, if the planner understands why the decision is for independence, the family will be able to ask for help if the plan does not work out.

Consider also this patient:

Nancy Riley has had COPD for 20 years. She had a lung removed for TB 30 years ago. Now at the age of 60 she has been diagnosed as having terminal cancer. She refuses all recommended therapy and wishes to go home to die. Her husband (the only family member in this country) does not wish to have his wife at home because he fears he cannot care for her. Family funds are limited, medical insurance coverage is poor, and neither spouse seems willing to change his or her position.

You will need to know much more about Mr. and Mrs. Riley's feelings, relationships, fears, and strengths to help each see what the other wants, fears, and can manage. Offers of support from home care, hospice, and pastoral care may help Mr. Riley to accept his wife's wish. On the other hand, he may not have accepted her death as imminent; that may be where help should begin. Do you know what her death will do to him? Is he frightened of the physical care? The loss of his wife? This is a situation where all the skills and strengths of the team involved in care will be needed. One of the two spouses will make the decision, and it is possible that no one will feel right about it. But the opportunity to be heard, to be counseled, and to see alternate plans will have been given.

These three illustrations point up the conflict for discharge planners and other health care professionals between what is thought to be good for the patient and what the patient chooses. The choice that is finally made will be difficult; it may be less than optimum and at times inappropriate.

Success or failure of the discharge plan should not be the criterion upon which the program or the concept of planning as an essential part of medical care is judged. Rather, one should see if the plan indeed "reflects both the patient's and family's internal and external social, emotional, medical and psychological needs and assets."[4]

chapter 6

human resources: roles and interdisciplinary relationships

The discharge planner needs to know the answers to the following questions:

- Who should administer the discharge planning program?

- How should administration support the program?

- Who should coordinate all the discharge planning functions carried out by the various health care professionals and agencies?

- Which disciplines and department should have major responsibility for discharge planning?

- What are the qualifications and functions of a discharge planning coordinator?

- Is a multidisciplinary approach to discharge planning appropriate?

- What other professionals, besides nurses and social workers, usually do discharge planning?

- What role does the physician play?

- What role does the department of nursing play?

- What role does the public health nurse coordinator or liaison play?

WHO SHOULD ADMINISTER THE PROGRAM OR HEAD THE DEPARTMENT?

To ensure that a patient's intra- and postinstitutional needs are met, a program based on the following ideas should be developed:

- Need for an interdisciplinary team approach.

- Conviction that continuity of care involves helping a patient with his nonmedical as well as medical needs.

- Philosophy that programs implemented by an institution are most likely to succeed when they are developed from within that institution.

The hospital or nursing home must officially integrate a discharge planning program into its total operation. Imprecise assignment of discharge planning responsibilities and haphazard supporting policies do not lead to the best patient care and the best utilization of limited resources. The hospital or nursing home must therefore have:

- Formal commitment to discharge planning with organized programs headed either by the administrator or a separate department responsible to administration.

- A designated health care professional with the ultimate authority and responsibility for discharge planning.

- Clear lines of responsibility and communication.

- Supporting policies and procedures.

- Competent staff members who understand their roles.

The Administrator

Many of the administrator's problems are in admission rather than discharge planning. However, the problems, resources, and facilities that bring a patient into the hospital or nursing home are the same ones that present difficulty at discharge planning time. Some of these are:

- The patient who wants to get into the institution but doesn't need to be there.

- The patient who does not want to go to the hospital but who, when he is ready for discharge, does not want to leave or go to another institution.

- Family pressure to admit or discharge a patient who has not been seen by the physician.

- The utilization review committee that believes that the patient should be discharged without a place to go, or that questions why he was initially admitted.

The administrator (assisted by the medical staff) should:

- Define the guidelines for the operation of the discharge planning process.

- Designate an individual who will be administratively responsible for the discharge program.

- Give full cooperation and approval to the program.

- Establish accountability for the program.

- Identify a central location for the collection of data and dissemination of information relevant to discharge planning.

The administrator has several options open for selecting an administrative structure:

- Assume administrative responsibility himself, assisted by a discharge planning coordinator.

- Delegate responsibility to a separate department that is equal to other departments.

- Assign a discharge planning coordinator who is directly responsible to administration or to the utilization review committee.

- Establish a multidisciplinary committee (with a designated chairperson) directly responsible to administration.

- Engage in a contractual agreement with an outside agency for a public health nurse to be responsible for the program.

- View the discharge planning program as one major component of the institution's quality assurance program.

THE DISCHARGE PLANNING COORDINATOR

More and more hospitals and nursing homes are designating one person to be accountable for development and operation of the discharge planning program. This person may also do daily discharge planning activities for individual patients, involving other health professionals in an interdisciplinary team approach. However, it is desirable to have a designated person (e.g., social worker or nurse) as the discharge planning coordinator, for when everyone is responsible, no one is responsible.

At the September 1984 annual conference, a special task force of the American Association for Continuity of Care delineated forces that assist or block interdisciplinary cooperation between professionals on the discharge team. Topmost among the principles agreed upon were the following:

- The ultimate integrating force in discharge planning is the patient.

- There is no single universally applicable recipe for which profession should be in charge of the discharge planning process.

- Interaction and involvement among the various disciplines who participate in the discharge planning process . . . both formally through structures and informally through relationships and communications . . . are essential for resolving turf problems.[1]

The discharge planning coordinator should be a registered professional nurse, a qualified social worker, or appropriate health professional. He or she should have leadership ability and the ability to motivate others. He or she should also have, or be able to gain, the respect of the medical staff and administration and should demonstrate a capacity to relate well to patients, their families, and hospital and other agency personnel. Job knowledge and experience should include background in an administrative position and familiarity with the organization and functions of the related departments in the hospital as well as knowledge of community resources.

For the following reasons, the discharge planning coordinator should report directly to administration:

- The discharge planning coordinator is carrying out a delegated administrative responsibility.

- A discharge planning program requires the participation and cooperation of at least 10 departments. The discharge planning coordinator has the staff function of evaluating and monitoring their activities as they relate to the institutional discharge planning program and suggesting corrective action as necessary. He or she needs administrative support and department-head status to carry out this function.

- Administration must hear the concerns of discharge planning directly. If these are filtered through any other discipline (social service, nursing, etc.), there is a tendency for bias to creep in.

- A coordinated discharge planning program is an important administrative tool for effectively dealing with community relations and malpractice issues.[2]

The discharge coordinator should have a baccalaureate or higher degree and two years of clinical or health care experience. Orientation to community health service organization and operation is desirable. The public health nurse or social worker has been exposed to a knowledge of health, and should have the ability to coordinate, plan, communicate, and evaluate personal health services. This person should also be aggressive enough to discuss issues with nurses, social workers, and doctors to request that referrals be made.

The discharge planning coordinator is responsible for the complete discharge planning process and its implementation. The coordinator is responsible, directly or through delegation, for the delivery of efficient and effective discharge planning services. The discharge planning coordinator is expected to assume overall responsibility for the discharge planning process in the hospital; develop, implement, and monitor the use of high-risk screening protocols; coordinate all disciplines' efforts so a smooth interdisciplinary process of discharge planning occurs; coordinate timely processing of Medicaid applications with the credit office; coordinate the alternate care notification process with utilization review committee and social work department, so that social workers receive prompt notification of alternate care patient designations; coordinate discharge planning rounds on each patient care floor; and chair regular discharge planning committee meetings.[3]

INTERDISCIPLINARY APPROACH

Historically, discharge planning has been performed in hospitals through collaboration between health care workers of various disciplines as problems arose in planning the care of patients. Discharge planning is best accomplished by a multidisciplinary team that begins its assessment of the patient's needs and goals as soon as practical for each patient, sometimes even before hospital admission. Team membership will vary according to the patient's needs and goals and the institution's staff and resources and may include the physician, nurse, social worker, physical or occupational therapist, pharmacist, dietitian, speech therapist, or any other health professional involved in the patient's care. Some of these disciplines should have permanent representation on the discharge planning team; others require only consultative positions. However, one person should be designated as the coordinator for the overall process so that accountability and responsibility are established.

The discharge planning model in use at the Long Island College Hospital (LICH), Brooklyn, N.Y., utilizes an interdisciplinary process. The following is excerpted from a condensed version of their discharge planning model, which was developed by Philip E. Jacobs, Ph.D., coordinator of discharge planning and director of social work:

Discharge planning program description. The discharge planning program at LICH may be thought of as having four phases: screening and identification, assessment, plan development, and plan implementation.

- *Screening and identification.* All patients admitted to the hospital do not require help with discharge planning, but each one is assessed whether or not this assistance is needed. The process is started as soon as possible, preferably within three working days of admission.

- It is the responsibility of the social worker on the floor to review each chart at the time of admission to determine whether or not a referral for discharge planning has been made or is necessary. Screening and identification continues during the patient's stay as some conditions may not be identified within three working days.

- *Assessment.* If a patient requires discharge planning services, assessments of patients' strengths and weaknesses and service needs are made by social work, utilization review, home care, rehabilitation medicine, and physician and nursing staff. Assessments should be performed by the social worker and inserted in the patient's medical record within one week of admission.

- *Plan development.* During the patient's stay, plans are developed by the social worker for discharge, whenever possible involving the patient/family and/or physician. Patient progress is reviewed in response to medical treatment and also in response to discharge plans and weekly medical rounds he held on every medical floor.

- *Plan implementation.* A discharge plan is implemented when the patient's acute care is concluded. This includes discharge from the hospital and the provision of postdischarge services either in an institutional setting or at home with support. Social worker follows up as needed with patient's postdischarge plan identifying problems and/or gaps in service as needed. The patient/family receives information sufficient for their understanding for posthospital needs, so they participate in and assist with plan implementation.

Multidisciplinary approach: The nursing process in discharge planning. Discharge planning responsibilities of the primary nurse are as follows: assist the patient and family to cope with the disruptions caused by illness or disability, thereby identifying the potential discharge problems and/or needs; collaborate with physician, patient, and family to plan for the utilization of other disciplines within the hospital to meet the patient's discharge problems and/or needs; involve appropriate hospital disciplines needed to provide expertise in matching hospital and community resources to meet the patient's discharge problems and/or needs; ensure the successful transition of patient care from the hospital to another facility or the patient's home through early planning; provide the patient and family with knowledge and understanding of the patient's illness and the prescribed treatment by carrying out appropriate patient teaching.

Multidisciplinary approach: Social work participation in discharge planning. Referrals to social work are followed up by social work within three days of the referral as possible, with an assessment within seven days.

After a referral has been made, and the case-management system has provided for the opening of a case, the discharge planning process moves to assist with the patient's needs. During this phase, the social worker provides case work, group work, and patient/family counseling services to the family and significant others. The focus of these services is to provide support to the patient as the worker enables the patient and significant others to progress through the experience of hospitalization and posthospital planning for continuity of care. The challenge to the worker is to play a balanced role in order to meet best the needs of the patient as circumstances dictate. This requires sometimes favoring a clinical role, sometimes favoring an advocacy role, and sometimes favoring an administrative systems-oriented role. The worker must evaluate patient characteristics such as diagnosis, medication needs, age, functioning level, rehabilitation potential, psychosocial factors, financial limitations, and other special needs. The worker needs to be aware of the range of available aftercare services and must evaluate these, along with the multidisciplinary staff, during patient rounds in order to determine what services are most appropriate to the needs assessment. Services including institutionalization, home care programs, specific posthospital services, and other supportive services such as homemaker services, meals-on-wheels, and the like are considered.

The detection and assessment phases are followed by efforts to place and discharge the patient when acute care is no longer medically required. For many patients and significant others, the period of acute medical care precipitates intense family and personal conflicts relating to the aging process, the acceptance of human mortality, and the conflicting needs that parents, children, and grandparents frequently have. All of these conflicts may be addressed by the social worker.

Financial realities often pose what seem to be insuperable difficulties to patients and their family members as a result of acute medical care. The discharge planning social worker interprets public sources of assistance to patients and significant others so that they do not feel a sense of shame and inadequacy when they need to rely on these funding sources.

As physicians become increasingly specialized, there is a corresponding need for the hospital to provide the patient and significant others with a single staff person who can answer their many questions concerning acute care and the posthospital phase.

Multidisciplinary approach: Department of Rehabilitation Medicine participation in discharge planning. The treatment therapist consults with the social worker regarding appropriate discharges as necessary and documents patient physical progress, or lack thereof, in daily notes. In addition, the treating therapist attends rehabilitation rounds to assist in completing all necessary planning for discharge and disposition.

Multidisciplinary approach: Role of Utilization Review Department in discharge planning. The Department of Utilization Review screens each Medicare and Medicaid admission to LICH. The detection of patients in need of discharge planning occurs on the date after admission for these patients. The need for discharge planning may not be apparent at the time of admission but may be evident during the course of hospital stay.

Initiation of discharge planning activity by the Utilization Review Department is sometimes prompted by medical notes such as documentation that the family is unwilling to accept the patient at home, indication from medical record that some form of assistance or actual long-term placement after the hospital stay may be needed, change in condition or diagnosis, and no referral to discharge planning prior to change.

Multidisciplinary approach: Home care and discharge planning. The goal of the LICH discharge planning program is to assist patients to return to the least restrictive environment possible. The most desirable plan is for the patient to return home, and the Home Care Program frequently is instrumental in helping achieve this plan.

The home care nurses participate in the weekly discharge planning rounds held on all patient floors. During these meetings, the nurses are available to respond to questions from nursing, social work, and physician staff concerning the appropriateness of different patients for home care referral and the likely home-care needs of different patients. In this way, the option of home-care referral is considered as part of the overall discharge planning process.[4]

THE ROLE OF THE PHYSICIAN

Informed medical staff members are key people in the discharge planning process. Even though referrals may be initiated by other health professionals, plans for continuing care must be approved and medical orders signed by the physician. The physician's role includes:

- Comprehensive understanding of all those involved: the patient, family, hospital administration, social workers, nursing staff, dietitians, clergy, and representatives of available community services.

- Support for discharge planning activities and plans.

- Making available information about the patient and family that will facilitate discharge planning and allow it to proceed in an effective and organized manner.

- Awareness of continuity of care problems.

- Provision for a structured program for the care of patients. Lack of planning all too often makes the patient's recovery and readaptation to society virtually impossible.

Brookdale Hospital Medical Center, Brooklyn, New York, expects that the attending physician will do the following:

1. Provide the following documentation on the patient's record (and encourage the house staff to do the same):

    a. The discharge plan on admission, with updates as necessary.

    b. Inclusion of discharge instructions and postdischarge plan in the discharge note (e.g., medications to be taken after discharge, diet, treatments and follow-up medical supervision).

2. Recognize that discharge planning requires communication and coordination with the inter-disciplinary health team; therefore:

   a. Refer the patient to the Discharge Planning Department when it is anticipated that the patient will require posthospital care (beyond follow-up with the physician).

   b. Use the physician's order sheet as a means of referring the patient to appropriate departments for assistance with the discharge plan.

3. Fully complete the forms required for referral to alternate levels of care on a timely basis.

4. Communicate *intent* to discharge 24–48 hours in advance.

5. Give specific instructions to the head nurse and the patient as to where and when the patient is to go for follow-up treatment.[5]

THE ROLE OF THE NURSING DEPARTMENT

The person designated as discharge planner cannot function effectively without nursing support. The chief nursing executive should:

- Promote an understanding of the requirements and goals of the program.

- Provide leadership and involvement to ensure continuity of patient care. Discharge problems and procedures should be standard items on the staff conference agenda.

- Require that written discharge policies and procedures be available to all staff.

- Provide for a member of the nursing staff to assume responsibility for (1) evaluation of the nursing referral system, (2) development of educational sessions on discharge planning, and (3) function as a liaison with the administration of the facility's discharge planning service.

Supervisor, charge, and staff nurses should be encouraged to provide continuing education to patients on their units about discharge planning. This includes the use of referrals. Something is wrong if the professional staff nurses are not making referrals and student nurses are. All personnel must share a strong conviction that the system is necessary and must support those endeavoring to meet patient needs.

Staff nurses who care for patients directly are best able to assess their immediate and long-term needs. Discharge planning is an integral component of total patient care and should be a part of every patient care plan. It must begin at the time of admission and follow the patient through the progression of his health care. Nurses should evaluate each patient's total situation. Merely considering the patient's diagnosis and the related discharge needs as bases for referral is insufficient. Discharge planning should be a part of everyday care of the patient.

THE ROLE OF THE PUBLIC HEALTH NURSE

The public health nurse is being used for discharge planning with increasing frequency. Hospitals may contract with a visiting nurse association or similar agency to place public health nurses in their facility. The nurse remains an employee of the agency while the hospital pays for the time she spends there.

Hospital administrators are also contracting with public health nurses from the local health department. The nurse usually works in the hospital part time until the number of referrals is too large to be handled by a part-time staff person. A public health nurse in a hospital works closely with the director of nursing and staff nurses, making rounds to locate patients who may need help with a sound discharge plan. All potential referrals are discussed with the patient's physician and plans are worked out jointly with the medical staff, nursing staff, and the patient. In this way, physicians and hospital staff nurses become familiar with the kinds of patients who need the public health nurse's attention. She functions as the planning discharge coordinator or liaison nurse between the hospital and the community.

In addition, some patients and their families are overwhelmed by the prospect of a nursing home or home care. Discussion with the public health nurse helps them adjust to the new environment and carry out the medical and treatment plans. When problems are identified early, serious ones may be averted and adjustment to the change from a dependent hospital role to a more independent one may be made more easily. If a skilled nursing home or home for the aged is recommended for the patient, the social service worker can be contacted to evaluate the possible choices and counsel the patient and family about transfer, adjustment, medical assistance programs, and the like.

A public health or home health nurse can visit the patient's home before he is discharged and answer the family's questions and offer suggestions (e.g., for the rearrangement of the physical setting in the home if the patient is handicapped). If the physician has ordered physical therapy, the public health nurse can make the proper arrangements. She has skills to make special adaptations in the home for the elderly patient who has a physical problem and is disoriented in the hospital but well oriented at home. She can carry professional nursing instruction and support to the family that prefers to have a family member at home through a difficult final illness, and she can provide important service to the young child who should be spared a prolonged separation from his family.

THE ROLE OF THE SOCIAL SERVICE WORKER

Social workers have always had discharge planning as one of their services. Because of the importance of the family in home care, a social evaluation of the strengths and weaknesses of family relationships is essential to discharge planning (e.g., the screening that precedes admittance of a patient to a home care setting). A continuous assessment of the impact of the program on the family is essential.

In addition to the medical history, the social history is of value in understanding the patient's background and in determining how he can be helped to adjust to his new surroundings. Individuals of different educational backgrounds, socioeconomic groups, ethnic and religious groups, and internal domestic situations respond differently in hospital and nursing home settings.

THE ROLE OF OTHER HEALTH PROFESSIONALS

Any health professional who assists in patient care has some contribution to make to the discharge planning process. Many disciplines should be involved in discharge planning. The support of the medical staff is crucial to getting a discharge planning program underway and to reaching the patients who need it. Key members of the medical, nursing, and administrative staff should be included in all planning. In each unit, regular conferences should be held in which the full range of professional staff departments are represented. At these meetings, the status of each patient should be evaluated and a total assessment arrived at relative to progress toward discharge.

chapter 7

program design: components and coordination

The person responsible for submitting a program plan to the administration and medical staff should find the answers to these questions:

- What existing organizational resources can be used to design a suitable program?

- Who should be included in the initial planning phase?

- Should special committees be established? If so, how should they function?

- What are the objectives of a coordinated discharge planning program?

- Will a pilot study be beneficial?

- How can an individualized discharge plan be established?

- How can the discharge planning activities performed by the various departments be integrated into a coordinated system, whether in the hospital, nursing home, or ambulatory care center?

- Should patient education be an integral part of the program?

- How do you write a discharge instruction sheet for the patient and family?

- What should be the focus of program evaluation?

Discharge planning requires commitment from the board of trustees and necessitates administrative planning and adequate numbers of staff. Each institution has different resources and needs and organizes its resources differently. The specific kind of coordinated program developed by a health institution will depend upon many factors, some of which are:

- The board's commitment to continuity of care.
- The characteristics of the patient population.
- The character of the facility (specific size, census, etc.).
- Sources of admissions (e.g., the whole state or one small area).
- Length of stay and other utilization patterns.
- Size and character of the surrounding community.
- Sources of available financing for patients and the institution.
- Types and numbers of personnel available.
- Composition of the medical staff.
- Educational needs of the staff and patients.

A strong building requires a well-designed foundation. Therefore, these initial steps should be taken in planning the program:

- Representatives of participating community agencies and groups should be invited to serve on an advisory ad hoc planning committee. This committee may continue to function in a planning and evaluating capacity after the program is implemented.

- Sources of funding should be identified (money for staff, office space, and the like; money for facilitating individual patients' discharges and associated educational efforts).

- Department heads and members of the medical, nursing, social work, and administrative staffs should be included in all discharge planning activities.

- Useful consultation can be obtained from the American Hospital Association, state hospital and nursing home associations, state departments of mental and public health, visiting nurse associations, home health care agencies, professional organizations such as the National League for Nursing and the Society for Hospital Social Work, and directors of local hospitals and nursing homes with established programs. (See pages 95–96.)

- Research the available literature. There are a variety of texts, booklets, pamphlets, and published guidelines on discharge planning. Publications such as *The Coordinator*, a trade magazine published by Coordinator Publications, Inc., and the American Hospital Association's *Discharge Planning Update* have published recommendations for problem solving and the development of discharge planning models. (See pages 87–93.)

- Visit social service departments and discharge planners at other hospitals or nursing homes to share materials and ideas and discuss problems and issues.

- The American Association for Continuity of Care has an annual conference with general sessions and workshops for discharge planners and home care professionals. They also publish periodic reports.

- An internal advisory committee, with representatives from medicine, nursing, social service, pharmacy, etc., may be set up to provide continuous guidance.

- The utilization review committee and quality assurance program coordinator should be fully informed of program planning and progress.

- The administrative structure for the program should be identified and established.

PROGRAM BUILDING BLOCKS

Decisions about the planning process will have to be made: How is it done? Who are the relevant staff members? For example, the *how* may be answered (depending on the phase of planning) by a staff conference, patient interviews, a case conference, analysis of each objective, use of consultants, feedback from community agencies, informal evaluation, and the like. The *who* involves the patients, their families, medical record analyst, discharge planning program staff, education specialist, and other relevant staff members.

Gain administrative support and establish lines of communication with the:

- Medical staff and utilization committee.
- Board of trustees or other appropriate persons.
- Department heads.
- Community agencies (e.g., transfer agreements between facilities).

Assess and select the patient population to be served, such as:

- New admissions.
- Repeat admissions for the same condition.
- Long-stay cases.
- Emergency room patients admitted for primary care.
- Patients transferred between units (e.g., skilled care to intermediate care, or intensive care unit to general ward).
- Posthospital home care or long term care candidates.

Assess levels of care that produce patients with special planning needs:

- Transfers between units and to other facilities
- Skilled nursing home patients to nonskilled status, day care, or other alternatives.

Write objectives that are functional, measurable, and realistic in terms of:

- Patient and family needs (both acute and chronic).
- Staff responsibilities and educational needs.
- Administrative functions and operation.
- Funds needed and cost benefits envisioned.
- Desirable utilization patterns.
- Patient educational needs (if patient education is not a separate program).
- General purpose and goals of the facility.
- Licensing and accreditation demands.
- Community resources to be used.
- Usual medical practices.
- Coordination of discharge goals established by other departments.
- Methods of disseminating information about the program.

Specific discharge planning program objectives must relate to an overall objective: to *focus first on the needs of the patient and then make provision for his optimum well-being, whether in the hospital, nursing home, physician's office, or in his own home.*

Select staff, assign responsibilities, write job descriptions, and orient staff, considering:

- Staff members' ongoing inservice education needs.

- Periodic multidiscipline, multifacility meetings to exchange ideas.

Develop operational policies, procedures, and methods. For example:

- Establish communication systems within the facility and between the facility and the community.

- Devise appropriate forms.

- Compile a policies and procedures manual.

- Maintain resource files.

- Plan a facilitywide patient education program, if needed.

- Select documentation methods and define areas of concern.

- Design method and process of evaluation.

Conduct a pilot study on an individual medical-surgical unit prior to hospitalwide implementation in order to:

- Identify and resolve problems.

- Evaluate effectiveness of data collection and retrieval.

- Determine if methods used to achieve objectives are appropriate, effective, and efficient.

- Evaluate patient and family response.

- Determine if patient discharge planning and teaching needs have been met.

- Conduct time and cost studies.

Carry out and concurrently evaluate the program; revise objectives, policies, and general operational format as needed.

HOW CAN AN INDIVIDUALIZED DISCHARGE PLAN BE ESTABLISHED?

The problem-solving steps that are necessary for creating a discharge and admission plan for an individual patient are similar to the phases involved in establishing a facilitywide discharge planning program. Primary emphasis must be placed on an understanding of who the patient is and what his needs are.

The American Hospital Association recommends that development of a discharge plan include the results of the assessment; the self-care instructions; and information from the patient, the family, and all relevant health care professionals. The discharge planner determines what services the patient needs, what options are available for providing them, and the patient and family are helped to understand the consequences of whatever plan they choose to adopt. A supportive climate is critical to appropriate decision making.[1]

Discharge plans may be totally individualized. As an alternative, standardized plans that allow for documentation of the unique characteristics of each patient may be used. The use of standardized plans, at least for patients who fall into major categories, is cost effective and ensures compliance with the institution's standards and goals.[2] Whichever type of plan is chosen, it must be:

- Realistic
- Functional
- Flexible
- Obtainable
- Efficient
- Effective
- Economical
- Organized
- Productive.[3]

The family's involvement or lack of involvement must also be considered. Health care facilities must guard against the depersonalization of patients, and a good discharge planning program helps to do this. Creating an individualized discharge or admission plan involves many factors simultaneously:[4]

- Involving the patient in as much decision making as possible.
- Determining the necessary level of postdischarge care (e.g., using Medicare and Medicaid's definitions of covered care).
- Determining what facility can best accommodate the patient at the required level of care.
- Arranging for the patient to be transported there.
- Initiating necessary patient education.
- Discovering the family and patient's wishes.
- Collaborating with key professionals.
- Deciding on equipment needs.
- Informing the family and patient as early as possible of what is to be expected after discharge.
- Finding funds to pay the bill.
- Deciding, if the patient is in a home care setting, if the more intensive services of the hospital or nursing home are needed.

As the patient enters the hospital, nursing home, or other facility, there are some essential planning steps.

Learn the Facts on Admission

Data on the patient's needs must be collected and recorded. Members of each professional discipline will need to gather facts to assist them in making a contribution to the total therapeutic regime, including the discharge plan. If sufficient time and effort are spent in developing an effective system of interdisciplinary record keeping and designing forms that are universally acceptable, both discharge planning and interdisciplinary and interagency communication will be enhanced.

An information sheet that can be used by all agencies involved in the institution's discharge planning process is the ideal. At a minimum, an interview guide should include:

- Home situation, present illness.

- Occupation.

- Education.

- Sociocultural background.

- Interests.

- Habits.

- Previous hospitalizations or home care.

- Expectations of this hospital or nursing home staff.

- Patient's adjustment to illness.

- Patient's expectations for discharge.

Make the Family Background an Inherent Part of the Recorded Admission Data

An understanding of the patient's background is essential in providing effective continuity of care. In regard to the patient's family, it has been found that acute and terminal illness are far more acceptable than chronic illness. In chronic illness, the length of time that family members must be involved is uncertain and their adjustments are varied. Studies show that family members have difficulty accepting a patient whose ambulatory status changes; thus a patient in a wheelchair is often less acceptable than a bedridden patient. Studies show that chronic illness in the young can be tolerated and accepted by families much more readily than it can in the aged.

The patient's mental state also needs consideration. Many individuals are admitted to the hospital or nursing home in a state of panic or confusion. While young people recover rapidly, an elderly person may remain confused for a long time, especially after a surgical or emergency procedure or transfer.

Know Where the Patient Came From

It is important to know where the patient came from immediately before admission to the institution, particularly for nursing home patients. For example, many patients list their landlady or public guardian as the person to be notified in case of an emergency. Such conditions affect the plans made for the patient's return home. Many home care programs depend on a reliable family member or friend to carry out procedures and assist in the treatment regimen between visits of health care personnel. Also, the patient's ethnic and religious background will affect his return home (e.g., the diabetic patient on a special diet may return to a home where proper food will not be prepared because of cultural or religious beliefs).

At Silver Cross Hospital in Joliet, Illinois, a continuity-of-care referral form is placed on the patient's chart by the discharge planning nurse or member of the discharge planning team. The referral form is used by all health team members. This form communicates the patient's needs and thus helps health professionals in the community to give continued care to the patient on discharge from the hospital. All referrals are completed before the patient's discharge, with physician's orders and signature and nursing care information. A supplemental form, which is attached, is a written plan used by the health team members to provide additional information from other departments (social services, dietary, physical therapy, and so on). A blank supplemental sheet is also sent to the agency or institution so that feedback information can be returned to the hospital and posted for health team members. The transfer information is telephoned to the agency or institution before the form is mailed by the discharge planning nurse. Copies are sent to the agency or institution, the medical records department, the physician, and the continuity of care office (see Appendix C).[5]

COORDINATION AND COMMUNICATION

There must be a high level of communication among all health professionals involved in discharge planning. For example, communication between the various shifts of hospital personnel who see the patient at different times of the day and observe him under different conditions is important.

Long Island College Hospital, in Brooklyn, New York, uses a discharge planning log to enhance communication. In a large teaching complex such as Long Island College Hospital (LICH), there is a need for a central written document through which various professionals working during various shifts can communicate with one another concerning discharge planning activities on behalf of patients. To meet this need, there is a discharge planning log on each patient care unit. The discharge planning log contains the following information: date of referral, person making the referral, patient's room number, and name and item requested. Nursing staff and the social work discharge planner must check the discharge planning log daily.[6]

PATIENT EDUCATION

An essential component of hospital, nursing home, home care, and ambulatory care service is patient education. A facility may include this service in the discharge planning program or have an entire department responsible for patient education.

An excellent resource for information on the development of patient and family education programs is the American Hospital Association, Center for Health Promotion, 840 North Lake Shore Drive, Chicago, Illinois 60611. The Association publishes a list of institutions recognized for outstanding achievement in the management of patient and family education programs.

The Discharge Instruction Sheet

It has been found that at discharge time the patient and his family are more anxious than usual, and verbal instructions alone are not adequate. Therefore, a written discharge instruction sheet should be given to each patient.

This is especially important for the patient who is discharged to self-care at home. Preprinted instruction sheets or computer-generated posthospital care plans that contain space for individualized information are time saving and economical and ensure that the patient receives the necessary instructions (see Appendix C). Instruction sheets should include:

- A brief description of the patient's diagnosis.

- Prescribed activity level.

- Medication list.

- Diet instructions.

- Other special instructions.

- Medical follow-up: what to do in an emergency, return appointments.

- Social and psychological instructions (if needed).

PROGRAM EVALUATION

Mechanisms should be established that will ensure continuous and thorough concurrent and retrospective review of the discharge planning program. Oakwood Hospital, Dearborn, Michigan, supports an evaluation method that includes the following factors:

- Appropriateness of care, referrals, transfers, and lengths of stay.
- Transfer rates to home care, nursing homes, and other hospitals.
- Planning and assessment needs met or unmet identified.
- Staff acceptance of the program.
- Feedback from other facilities.
- Utilization of services.
- Patient and family satisfaction with services provided.[7]

Information should be elicited from patients, families, and health professionals in facilities that receive the discharged patients. This may be accomplished via telephone contact, post cards, or questionnaires.

chapter 8

documentation

Garnett Jones

What are the puposes of documentation in discharge planning?

- To communicate to all health care team members the current status of the patient's discharge plan.

- To provide a permanent record of the services received by the patient and the role of each discipline in providing them.

- To provide a record of patient case management.

- To provide information for regulatory and accreditation reviews.

- To provide an educational tool for staff training.

- To provide data for audit, quality assurance, and statistical analyses.

- To create a permanent record for legal puposes.

GENERAL PRINCIPLES OF DOCUMENTATION IN DISCHARGE PLANNING

- Documentation should reflect the entire discharge planning process.

- The patient's medical record should reflect the progress of the patient's discharge plan from admission to discharge.

- There should be a common source document, usually progress notes or a special discharge planning form; any recording of pertinent information in a location other than the patient's record should include a notation to that effect on the common source document.

- The documentation should reflect the involvement of all persons participating in the discharge planning process: the patient and significant others, the physician, and other members of the health care team.

- All documentation should be specific, including names of persons, facilities, products, and health care providers, patient needs, and levels of care.

- Discharge planning activities should be documented as they occur, or, at a minimum, summarized every seven days.

- Documentation should show what information has been provided to the patient.

- When a patient or family member chooses a plan for care after discharge that is considered by a health team member to be inappropriate, documentation should show that the patient or family member and other involved members of the health team have been so informed.

- Documentation of patient education should describe the information that was presented and any evidence that the patient comprehended the instruction. Detailed instructions and protocols need not be documented in full if sample copies are on file in the medical records department.

- Documentation should reflect any referrals to other health care professionals for consultation regarding discharge planning.

- Health care professionals who receive a referral for consultation in discharge planning should, within 24–48 working hours, document the date and source of referral, any action taken, and tentative plans for follow-up.

- There should be a discharge summary, showing the final discharge plan, with the signature of the health care professional who is responsible for coordinating the plan.

- An appropriate summary should be provided to those responsible for the patient's postdischarge care.

- A copy of any interagency referral should be included in the patient's permanent record.

- The person responsible for coordinating the hospital discharge planning program should participate in the hospital's monitoring of the timeliness and appropriateness of discharge planning documentation, using the standards of the health care setting.

- There should be documentation of the effectiveness of the discharge planning process.

DOCUMENTATION BY STAFF NURSES

Documentation of the nursing process should include discharge planning from admission to discharge and should be individualized to the patient.

The Initial Nursing Assessment

Data should be collected that helps the nurse begin to do anticipatory planning for care following discharge and should address the patient's:

- Perception of his or her health status and reason for admission.

- Pattern of managing his or her own health care.

- Recent utilization of the health care system and community resources.

- Tentative plan for care after discharge (residence, caregivers, transportation).

- Any self-care deficits that may affect postdischarge care: functional limitations, medical impairments, health risk factors, psychosocial and economic concerns.

- Occupation, education, spiritual, and cultural/ethnic factors.

The Nursing Care Plan

Documentation on the nursing care plan should include:

- A brief statement about the tentative plans for after discharge that is current and correlated with the plans of the patient and family.

- Discharge planning problems, or any self-care deficits that will persist after discharge. These may be related to the illness or injury or limited financial resources.

- Planned nursing actions that address the self-care deficits that may persist after discharge. These may include nursing measures, referrals to or consultation with other health care professionals, referrals to community resources, or investigation or advocacy.

- Goals that are mutually set by the patient and nurse in planning for postdischarge care.

- Evaluation of the results of the nursing actions, which may or may not indicate the need for additional actions to be taken before discharge to meet the patient's needs following discharge.

The Nurse's Progress Notes

Documentation of discharge planning activities by the staff nurse should follow the general principles of documentation in discharge planning when appropriate.
Additional considerations for the staff nurse include the following:

- The patient's needs as related to discharge planning should be documented, even when no solutions are available.

- Duplication should be avoided. The nurse does not need to describe discharge planning problems or actions being addressed by other members of the health care team. Document only what is pertinent.

- Don't enter the same information in several places.

THE DISCHARGE SUMMARY

The staff nurse should document on the discharge summary what is appropriate within the standards and guidelines of the health care setting. The signature of the staff nurse on the discharge summary shows responsibility for the coordination of the entire discharge plan. The nurse may or may not be responsible for documenting the final discharge plan of other health care professionals on the patient's discharge summary.
See Appendix C for sample discharge planning record forms.

quality assurance

Jo Keblusek

The discharge planner should ask:

- What is quality assurance?

- What minimum data should be collected routinely on each patient?

- What are the essential components of a discharge planning quality assurance program?

- What factors should be monitored?

- What are some possible indicators of high risk?

- Can readmissions become a problem? When? Why?

WHAT IS QUALITY ASSURANCE?

Quality assurance is a systematic, continuous set of activities carried out to ensure, or improve, the quality of care. The purposes of these activities include:

- Identification of important elements of care.

- Assessment of services provided.

- Determination of compliance with acceptable standards.

- Identification of deficiencies and problems.

● Implementation of corrective action.

● Monitoring of results.

In a hospital it is essential that the discharge planning quality assurance program be part of the hospital's overall quality assurance program. Many issues and concerns are common to many departments and require a system of communication which transcends these boundaries for resolution.

WHAT ARE THE ESSENTIAL COMPONENTS OF A DISCHARGE PLANNING QUALITY ASSURANCE PROGRAM?

A complete quality assurance program has three essential components:

● Data collection system.

● Organized system of evaluation (peer review).

● Patient identification and access system.

Data Collection

Every discharge planning program should include a method of routinely collecting patient information. Ideally, statistics should be computerized and tied to the patient's hospital number. However, if computer access is not available, a manual collection system is necessary.

Data to be collected routinely on each patient should include, at a minimum:

● Social characteristics (age, living arrangements, financial classification).

● Discharge planning service provided (screening, assessment, arrangement of services).

● Problems identified.

● Disposition (services arranged) and outcome.

A complete data collection system provides essential information and quick access to those patients to be included as a sample in a particular monitoring topic, such as a review of discharges to nursing homes. A computer run of all cases discharged to a nursing home will provide the ages of patients who received this service, the amount and kind of discharge planning services given, and expected outcomes.

System of Evaluation (Peer Review)

All major aspects of discharge planning should have stated elements and standards of service. A general procedure for discharge planning may be followed, or there may be specific procedures for various diagnoses or dispositions.

The discharge planners must assist in the development of a set of criteria for adequate care and must, as providers, agree that the elements are necessary for adequate care. Once consensus is reached, the criteria are compared with actual discharge planning activities.

Patient Identification and Access

Discharge planners should have early and automatic access to all patients identified as potentially needing their service. High-risk criteria for discharge planning should be applied on admission to alert the discharge planner to patients needing screening and assessment. A screening mechanism should be in place to facilitate this casefinding upon admission.

High-risk criteria vary between hospitals and within hospitals. However, at the very least, high-risk indicators should include:

- Patients admitted from another institution.
- Patients with no known relatives.
- Patients recently discharged from a hospital.
- Patients with terminal illness.
- Trauma victims.
- Patients with diagnosis of CVA or related condition.
- Patients with chronic or debilitating conditions.
- Patients beyond a certain predetermined age.
- Patients who live alone.
- Patients with inadequate resources.
- Patients with no known residence.

Each hospital must develop its own list of indicators based on individual past experience.

WHAT FACTORS SHOULD BE MONITORED?

Whatever is important to the delivery of quality discharge planning should be continuously monitored. Mandates for ongoing review can be found in

- Peer review organization requirements.
- JCAH regulations.
- Discharge planning policy and procedure manuals.
- Hospital policies.

Quality assurance monitoring may be

- **Continuous:** to ensure consistency and to identify problems as they occur.
- **Short-term:** to focus on isolated problems until resolution.
- **Concurrent:** to review cases of current patients.
- **Retrospective:** to review cases of discharged patients.

Which method is used depends on the purpose and intent of the review. A restrospective review is most often used to evaluate a given service or to determine the cause of a problem. Most quality assurance monitoring is retrospective.

A concurrent review can be carried out to prevent a potential problem from occurring or to determine compliance when corrective action has been defined. An example of concurrent review follows:

- **Problem:** ongoing monitoring of patients with diagnosis of CVA and extended length of stay indicated delay in or absence of discharge planning screenings.
- **Corrective action:** to screen all CVA patients within 24 hours of admission.

● **Concurrent review:** of all CVA cases within 48 hours of admission to determine whether corrective action has been carried out.

Monitoring may be:

● **Process oriented:** the focus of the review is on procedure and on compliance with procedures.

● **Outcome oriented:** the focus of the reviews is on final results, such as improved social functioning, maintenance or improvement of health, goal attainment. This type of review is highly desirable but also highly subjective.

Suggested topics for monitoring include

● Delayed discharges.

● Readmissions within a specified number of days.

● Discharges to skilled nursing facilities.

● Referrals to home health care.

● Patient satisfaction.

● Compliance with specific discharge planning protocol.

● Timeliness of service.

● Transfers.

An example of a discharge planning monitor that is continuous, retrospective, and process oriented follows. It embodies all the previously discussed components: data-collection system, peer-review system, patient identification and accessibility, and computer accessibility.

Topic: 14-Day Readmissions

● **Problem:** patients readmitted to the hospital within 14 days of discharge may pose a reimbursement problem. The utilization review committee reviews the readmissions for medical necessity as well as intensity of service.

● **Purpose:** to review records of all patients readmitted to the hospital within 14 days of discharge to evaluate:

1. Preadmission screening.

2. Appropriateness of discharge planning.

3. Whether the discharge plan was implemented.

4. The reason for readmission.

5. Whether discharge planning was initiated after readmission.

● **Data needed:** computer printout showing all patients readmitted within 14 days of discharge for previous quarter. Information should include patient's identification number, dates of both admissions, whether discharge planning was done, and which discharge planner was involved.

● **Procedure:** *Phase 1*—Review all cases that did not receive discharge planning services to determine:

1. Whether patient should have received discharge planning services. If yes, what corrective action is needed to prevent recurrence of problem?

TABLE 1. MONITORING OF 14-DAY READMISSIONS.

Hospital Record Number	120	230	470	810	360	392	501
Discharge Planner Number	*1*	*3*	*2*	*3*	*1*	*2*	*1*
Element							
1. Patient/family perception of posthospital needs	√	√	√	√	0	√	√
2. Patient status preadmission							
a. Mental	0	√	0	0	0	0	0
b. Physical	0	√	√	√	0	√	0
c. Living arrangements	0	√	√	√	0	√	0
d. Financial	0	√	√	√	0	√	0
3. Current condition	√	√	√	√	√	√	√
4. Anticipated status at discharge includes							
a. deterioration/change in #2 above	0	√	0	√	0	0	0
b. collaboration with medical staff	√	√	√	√	√	√	√
c. existing assistance	√	√	√	√	√	√	√
5. Services indicated (home care, equipment, placement)	√	√	√	√	√	0	√
6. Actions to be taken to provide needed services, referrals, or arrangements	√	√	X	√	√	√	X
Total number of deficiencies	5	—	2	1	6	3	5

√ = Evident in medical record
0 = Deficient in medical record
X = Justified deficiency (patient refused, unable to be interviewed, etc.)

2. Whether readmission could have been prevented with (improved) discharge planning.

• *Phase 2*—Review all cases that did receive discharge planning to determine compliance with established protocol. See Table 1: The left column lists the discharge planning protocols developed with and accepted by the discharge planners as elements of quality care. All records are reviewed for evidence that these elements were addressed. In the development of these protocols, acceptable exceptions were also identified, such as a patient's inability to be interviewed, nonavailability of family, and a patient's refusal of service. On completion of review, the worksheet is analyzed for results and recommendations. These are summarized in Table 2, which shows that discharge planner 1 had 16 deficiencies out of a possible 33 (48% com-

TABLE 2. RESULTS AND RECOMMENDATIONS.

	Results/Findings	*Recommendations/Follow-up*
Element		
1	86% compliance (one deficient record)	
2a	86% noncompliance	In-service program will be provided to all staff members on (date).
2b	57% compliance	All deficiencies in elements 2b, 2c, and 2d involved
2c	57% compliance	discharge planner #1. Discharge planner #1 will be
2d	57% compliance	supervised in this area; cases will be reviewed concurrently until compliance is achieved.
3	Full compliance	
4a	71% compliance	Cases will be reviewed with discharge planners 1 and 2.
4b	Full compliance	
4c	Full compliance	
5	86% compliance	
6	Full compliance	

pliance). These results are consistent with previous performance reviews. A performance review is scheduled. Cases #120, #360, and #501 received inadequate discharge planning. In addition, for elements 2a and 4a criteria will be reviewed with all staff members at a staff meeting, and all cases will be reviewed concurrently. Finally, monitoring of all cases will continue and a report will be made to the quality assurance committee at the end of the next quarter.

A monitor such as this shows where discharge planning was appropriate and where it was deficient. It identifies the specific areas in which deficiencies occurred and pinpoints who was involved. Monitoring provides topics for staff inservice education program needs and is a tool for evaluating staff productivity and performance. In short, quality assurance monitoring isolates a problem, recommends corrective action, and allows for continuation of review to determine compliance and sustained improvement. An ongoing quality assurance program promotes quality service, professionalism, efficiency, productivity, and accountability.

Part III
TOPICS IN DISCHARGE PLANNING

chapter 10

the Georgia Baptist Medical Center discharge planning model

Brenda C. Nave

This article describes the discharge planning program and department at Georgia Baptist Medical Center, a large urban hospital. Georgia Baptist Medical Center (GBMC) is a 523-bed teaching hospital and tertiary-care center in Atlanta, Georgia. GBMC believes that coordinated discharge planning is essential for maintaining high-quality patient care. Extra attention is currently focused on discharge planning because of increased emphasis on continuity of patient care and the monitoring of health care by regulatory agencies and third-party payers. Discharge planning is seen as a means of reducing length of stay and helping to control the increase of health care costs. However, this current interest must not detract from the basic operating philosophy that every patient has a right to quality discharge planning and that each patient must be recognized as an individual with unique needs for continuing health care.

Georgia Baptist Medical Center supports the multidisciplinary approach to discharge planning. We believe that discharge planning is everybody's business. But we thoroughly concur with the 1966 National League for Nursing "Statement on Continuity of Nursing Care," which states that "What's everybody's business is nobody's business . . . ." Responsibility for discharge planning must be assigned to someone. At GBMC it is assigned to the discharge planning department, which consists of five registered nurses, who function primarily as discharge planners or coordinators, plus one clerical support person. The assignment of nursing units is divided among the nurses so that each works with an average census of about 100 patients. The nursing unit assignment and census requires each nurse to activate or participate daily in discharge planning for approximately 15 to 20 patients whose posthospital needs require special discharge planning services. Staff nurses are responsible for giving discharge instructions to patients whose discharge is routine.

Discharge planning begins during the admission phase and continues with the patient and family as they progress through the hospitalization and health services to posthospital care. The discharge plan is initiated on admission, at the same time as the nursing care plan, and is modified to meet the patient's needs for continuing care.

The discharge planning department has several functions. First, it coordinates all the services of the health care team to ensure that patients and families have access to services after they are discharged. This coordinated action helps provide continuity of care. The department also creates awareness of the need for continuity of care among physicians and other hospital staff members by providing orientation and inservice education programs. Contacts are made with community health agencies so that they can be involved in the development of discharge plans. Third, the department uses all available resources to design a patient care plan that promotes self-help and self-care and reinforces patient education. Fourth, the department publicizes the process and the benefits of discharge planning through inservice programs, written reports, and educational programs for physicians, administrators, and department directors. Educating everyone about discharge planning is essential to our program. Finally, the department submits a monthly report to management and maintains statistics on all referrals and department activities. A file of information, including copies of all correspondence, is maintained on each patient.

Role of the Discharge Planning Nurse

The discharge planning nurse is a patient advocate. She identifies patients for whom discharge planning will involve more than routine procedures. Case finding includes daily rounds on each nursing unit to discuss with the nursing staff the anticipated needs of each patient. The risk factors include age, diagnosis, health status, nutritional status, and previous living arrangements; all are important in case finding. Admission and preadmission screening reviews for discharge planning are done when possible. Additional case finding includes information and referrals from utilization review coordinators, social workers, dietitians, therapists, and families.

Interviewing and counseling with the patients and their families is a primary part of developing a discharge plan. The discharge process involves *assessing* (getting the facts), *diagnosing* (what exactly does the patient need?), *planning* (when, where, for how long?), *implementing* (putting the plan in motion), *documenting* (recording in the medical record), and *evaluating* (follow-up from agencies, nursing homes, patients, and families).

The discharge planning nurse may make referrals to social workers, therapists, chaplains, patient education, nurses, and other specialists inside and outside the hospital. Discharge planning nurses work with social service staff in providing direct or consultant services to the patient and family for further development of continuity of care services.

The discharge planning nurse plans and sets up the referral to other facilities—hospitals, extended care facilities, intermediate care facilities, rehabilitation centers, personal care homes, and so forth. She coordinates pertinent information and correspondence and assists in completing the Georgia Baptist Medical Center transfer form (see Appendix C). Most of the forms used were designed by the discharge planning department for consistency and to eliminate confusion caused by use of many different agencies' forms. Copies of all referral forms are retained for the medical record and the discharge planning file. A Consent to Release Medical Records form is obtained before photocopying and sending the medical information requested by the receiving facility. Assistance is provided the physician for doctor's orders to be sent with the patient to the receiving facility. If needed, an ambulance transport form is completed for the ambulance service and for billing purposes (see Appendix C).

If the services of a home health agency are needed, the GBMC referral form to home health agencies is prepared for the visiting nurse, home health aide, physical therapist, speech therapist, or social worker.

The discharge planning nurse also prepares referrals for durable medical equipment and supplies. She works with doctors, therapists, nurses, equipment companies, and pharmacists to arrange appropriate equipment and supplies in the home. Volunteer and community organizations are brought into use, such as the American Cancer Society, the Diabetes Association, and church groups. Patient services to the terminally ill include hospice and facilities for terminal care.

The discharge planning nurse collaborates with the utilization review committee, physicians, and nurses to accomplish a timely patient discharge. Daily communication with utilization review is maintained. The discharge planning director is a member of the utilization review committee.

The discharge planning department is represented on the oncology committee, patient education committee, DRG task force, geriatric task force, and in nursing management. The discharge planner is a valuable resource person on the health and financial aspects of referrals to home care services and transfers to nursing homes.

The discharge planning office, located inside the hospital, is the focal point of formal discharge planning activities. The office contains a desk and telephone for each discharge planning nurse. Since the discharge planning nurse spends much of her time on the nursing units, an audio page system is used. Pages can be received from doctors, nurses, patients and families, agencies, and others. The office is a storehouse for reference material and information for discharge planning. Books, reports, articles, facility policies and guidelines are available for use by the discharge planning nurse or anyone else. Rehabilitation information and equipment catalogs are kept for reference. The office houses the community agency manuals, directories, and guides, as well as copies of pertinent federal and state regulations. An IBM personal computer with a commercial database program is used for logging patient information, referral data, and statistical information. An ongoing resource file is maintained to make contacts more efficient. Materials are provided to all departments for information and data about discharge planning.

chapter 11

an educator's perspective: discharge planning model

Lynda N. Brown
Barbara E. Brown

During this transitional phase of cost containment, DRGs, and PPOs, health care providers need to develop more creative approaches to health care delivery. The primary focus of this paper is to examine discharge planning from an educator's viewpoint. A brief look at the historical development of discharge planning is provided, as well as a definition of the concept. An overview and analysis of specific changes in the health care system that are altering nursing practice is presented. Also included are discussion of changing client characteristics and how these changes affect the client's family and community. In addition, a model for student learning about discharge planning is presented and utilized to design a transitional model for discharge planning for hospital nurses. The paper concludes by exploring some futuristic ideas.

HISTORICAL DEVELOPMENT

The need for discharge planning was recognized over a century ago. In 1885 Sir Charles Loch remarked,

> There is a clear need of someone at the hospital to direct the patient . . . to present those interests other than medical and harmonize them with the purely medical interests . . . . He should help to make those who can become self reliant so, and obtain help for those who need it. Without this, the medical care may fail of its good purpose.[1]

During the past hundred years the concept of discharge planning has been given many labels: convalescent care, after care, progressive patient care, follow-up care, and home care.[2] Nurses have been involved with this concept in the past and continue to be involved with this concept in the present. Moreover, our prediction for future nursing practice includes a more pronounced effort in discharge planning.

In recent years the concept of discharge planning has received support from the American Hospital Association. In the "Patient's Bill of Rights" there is a statement of interest:

> The patient has the right to expect reasonable continuity of care . . . . The patient has the right to expect that the hospital will provide a mechanism whereby he is informed by his physician or a delegate of his physician of the patient's continuing health requirements following discharge.[3]

Who this "delegate" was, however, was often left to chance. In the past when nurses discussed why discharge planning had not been completed, excuses included the following: we didn't know when the patient was leaving, we didn't know what we should teach, we didn't have sufficient time. But times have changed and nurses have begun to look at discharge planning from a different perspective.

ELEMENTS OF DISCHARGE PLANNING

There is an increasing need for nurses to assist patients in planning for their discharge. There is an expanding volume of literature on this topic. We have analyzed this literature to identify the main elements of the discharge planning process and its application, which include the following points:

1. Discharge planning begins at admission and is part of the nursing process.
2. Discharge planning is a holistic approach to health planning that ensures continuity of care.
3. Discharge planning is required for all patients.
4. Agencies should have a formal process for discharge planning.
5. The success of discharge planning is dependent on the identification of the patient needs and the resources to meet those needs.[4]

It is through the application of these elements that nurses can help clients achieve their highest level of functioning and wellness potential.

CHANGES IN THE HEALTH CARE SYSTEM

Home health care has finally been discovered by the mainstream of the traditional health care industry.[5] A number of factors have helped to catapult home health care into its rightful place in our society. High on the list are the changing nature of the elderly population, the need for high-technology medical devices in the home environment, the implementation of DRGs with the concomitant increase in the number of referrals, and the public's demand for less expensive and more humane alternatives to institutionalization.[6]

As educators, we feel the need to instill in student nurses a new commitment to meeting the challenge of delivering health care in the home. Nursing faculty must promote the development of the advanced skills needed to carry out this nursing role, which links hospital with the home. This requires a different knowledge base than our traditional areas of specialization, such as community health nursing and medical-surgical nursing. The new nurse specialist must be expert in a broader area. This nurse must be highly skilled in interpersonal communication and must be able to analyze Medicare and other third-party payment benefits, analyze agency potential and referral practices, and match these areas with the health needs of clients and families.

In our educational institutions, we need to concentrate student learning experiences in the community rather than in the hospital. The reasons for this radical change of focus include the declining hospital census, shortened length of hospital stay, and changing health care insurance plans.

MODEL FOR STUDENT LEARNING

Because of these changes in hospitalization, students' access to patients is limited. In order for student nurses to have quality learning experiences, creative approaches must be designed. One approach we developed and utilized with success is the patient follow-through approach to home care, an adaptation of a follow-through of a patient on an inpatient service in a hospital (for example, surgery or delivery). In this new approach to home care, the student provides acute nursing care in the home after the patient's discharge. The student learns to employ basic nursing skills in the home rather than in the hospital.

If this mode of treatment is used, patients demonstrate more independence in activities of daily living and become more self-care oriented. The patient's behavior is far different from that of the patient admitted to the hospital for total care. This change in the mode of treatment requires the student nurse to assess, plan, implement, and evaluate at a higher level than was previously required.

The nature of patient and family teaching has also changed, in that teaching has become a primary nursing role instead of the secondary role it was in the past. Patient and family teaching begins at admission and continues after discharge. Teaching must be incorporated into discharge planning when the patient enters the health care delivery system and must continue to be reinforced in the home by the student nurse.

TRANSITIONAL MODEL FOR HOSPITAL NURSES

The student model for patient follow-through may be applied to hospital staff nurses who wish to be retrained to provide care in the home. This model may provide some nurses with an alternative to staff termination when changes in the health care system result in lower inpatient census. Hospital nurses with acute-care skills may wish to take advantage of this opportunity for an alternative mode of providing care and bring their valuable skills to home health nursing.

FUTURISTIC IDEAS

It is obvious that the nature of the health care delivery system has changed and continues to change. Nursing must respond to this change through creative, innovative, and dynamic actions. In the educational preparation of nursing students and in continuing education for nurses who are caught in this dilemma of health care transition, nurse leaders need to assess, design, and implement new programs to meet these new challenges. If this is accomplished, nurses may be the people who are most successful at providing for the patient's needs for continuity of care.

Amidst all these changes in the health care delivery system, we believe that discharge planning is what holds the system together. Creative, innovative approaches to health care delivery are the means by which nurses can reach out to patients and families making the transition from hospital to home.

chapter 12

hospital discharge planning for continuity of care: the national perspective

John Feather
Linda O. Nichols

Hospital discharge planning for continuity of care is now recognized as critical for both acute care and long term care.* The financial viability of the hospital now depends in part on its ability to discharge patients quickly, and long term care facilities will continue to get most of their clients directly from hospital discharge planning. This interest is reflected in the growth of specialized publications for discharge planners and the creation of national organizations for these professionals.

Discharge planning has not always been such a prominent part of the health care system. It has traditionally been a low priority for hospitals, since the "real work" of patient care was seen as completed by the point of discharge, and only the final paperwork needed to be done for reimbursement. The task was often placed in the social work or nursing department for administrative convenience, rather than made a part of a well-developed plan for insuring the continuity of patient care.

This traditional lack of interest in discharge planning is reflected in the lack of systematic data available on it. Although a tremendous amount of information is collected about the health care system by government and private agencies, very little relates directly to discharge planning problems. This chapter is a report on the first national study to focus specifically on discharge planning. Although the data obtained are necessarily limited, they provide a statistically reliable picture of hospital discharge planning in the United States, including the effects of prospective payment using diagnosis related groups (DRGs) for Medicare reimbursement.

THE NEED FOR A NATIONAL STUDY

Most studies of discharge planning fall into one of three groups. The first, and by far the largest group, is studies of discharge planning at a single hospital.[1] These studies vary greatly in sophistication, but in general they report on how one hospital developed discharge planning procedures and how those procedures work. Studies belonging to the second group compare different hospitals in the same

*The authors would like to thank Suzanne Schultz and David Folts for their assistance in the research reported here.

community.[2] All of these studies concern hospitals in major cities (usually New York) and are often more descriptive than analytic. The third and smallest group of studies consists of reports on discharge planning nationally.[3] Although these studies add greatly to an overview of discharge planning, they have serious limitations. None use random sampling that would allow generalizability. Several focus on other issues (such as Medicare or home health care) and only touch on discharge planning in passing. Surveys using membership list of national organizations or magazine mailing lists overrepresent the most active and sophisticated discharge planners and often ignore part-time discharge planners in small or rural hospitals.

The limitations of past research create a need for a cross-community study based on a random sample of hospitals. Such a sample allows greater generalizability and thus provides a truer picture of hospital discharge planning across the United States. This need provided the rationale for the study reported in this chapter.

METHODOLOGY OF THE NATIONAL STUDY

This research is based on a national sample of 200 accredited U.S. hospitals drawn from the American Hospital Association listing; thus results are generalizable to all U.S. hospitals. The study was conducted in two phases. The first phase (time 1) gathered a great deal of general information about the discharge planning process and the hospital. The second (time 2), conducted a year later, focused on the changes caused by the introduction of DRGs.

Time 1

In 1983, the administrators of the 200 randomly selected hospitals were contacted and asked to identify all persons actively involved in discharge planning in the hospital. Some hospitals were inappropriate for the study (e.g., student health centers, prisons) and were eliminated from the sample. All identified discharge planning personnel were sent an extensive questionnaire along with an explanatory cover letter. The questionnaire was developed over the course of a year and can be divided into the following topics: general description of the discharge planning process; specific questions about the organization of discharge planning in the hospital; questions about the process itself; characteristics of the discharged patients; attitudinal questions about the quality of discharge planning; and characteristics of the respondent. The questionnaire took between 45 minutes and one hour to complete. Two complete follow-ups and a reminder postcard were sent to nonrespondents. The final response rate represented 72 percent of all eligible hospitals in the sample (238 individuals).

Data about characteristics of the hospital (e.g., size, staffing patterns, number of discharges) were obtained from the American Hospital Association. Each hospital was also matched with data from the 1980 U.S. Census on characteristics of its community.

Time 2

In July and August 1984, the respondents from the first phase of the study were recontacted and sent a questionnaire about the effects of the Medicare prospective payment system on discharge planning. Since a great deal of information had been gathered at time 1, the second questionnaire was shorter. Some questions were repeated at time 2 to measure changes, and additional questions specifically about DRGs were asked. Only those respondents whose hospitals were using DRGs for reimbursement were included in this phase; thus many respondents from time 1 were excluded. A total of 121 respondents are represented in time 2.

Limitations

Although this research is the first national study of discharge planning based on a generalizable sample, it has several limitations. The size of the sample is relatively small, and thus separate analyses cannot be conducted for different types of hospitals. In addition, some of the questions might have elicited different responses even for the same situation. The outcome measures used are subjective judgments by the discharge planners, rather than objective standards. However, used with some caution, the study results provide a reliable picture of discharge planning nationally.

DISCHARGE PLANNING CHARACTERISTICS

The hospitals in the sample vary greatly, as shown in Table 1. The average number of medical and surgical beds in these hospitals is 170, but that number ranges from 6 to 732 beds. Most hospitals (57%) were in urban areas, and many served communities with a higher percentage of elderly residents than the national average. Many hospitals had additional specialized services that affect discharge planning, including outpatient departments (47%), home health care (11%), skilled nursing facility (11%), and hospice (9%).

Almost half (38%) of the responding hospitals had part-time discharge planning teams, while 16% had full-time units whose sole responsibility was discharge planning. The interdisciplinary teams were usually composed of nurses and social workers, with physicians also present on about half of the teams. A member of the hospital administration was rarely present, but representatives from continuing care agencies were represented on about one-third of the teams.

Despite the dominance of the team model for discharge planning in the health care journals, this model has yet to be fully implemented in most U.S. hospitals. Many discharge planners work alone. One-third of hospitals reported that only one person was involved in discharge planning in the hospital, so that the isolated discharge planner is almost as common as the team.

For most respondents, discharge planning is only one part of their duties. These include patient care (for nurses), counseling (for social workers), utilization review, and administration. Some do not even have discharge planning as part of their written job description (15%). Some of these responsibilities enhance discharge planning by giving the planner greater knowledge of the patient, but some are conflicting roles. On average, our respondents spend half of their time each week on discharge planning.

The hospitals in our sample processed an average of 35 patients per month through discharge planning, but once again the range is wide, from 1 patient to 250 per month. Planning generally begins

TABLE 1. NUMBER OF HOSPITALS IN SAMPLE BY TYPE.

Type	Number
Not for profit	
State	4
County	7
City	5
City/County	2
Hospital District	13
Church	11
Other Not for Profit	59
Profit	
Partnership	2
Corporation	13
Military	5
Veterans	3
TOTAL	124

within four days of admission. In an average month, 10 patients leave the hospital before all continuing care arrangements are made; in an average week, 6 patients are being held in the hospital because a nursing home bed cannot be found.

Professionally, one-half of discharge planners are social workers, one-quarter are nurses, and the rest are from other educational backgrounds. Most have held their job five years or less, while one-third have had jobs with other agencies concerned with discharge planning (e.g., nursing homes, state agencies). Most (66%) maintain ties with their discipline through membership in professional organizations or through subscription to professional journals. Nine percent have been involved in political action to change legislation concerning discharge planning, although this percentage may increase with the rise of national organizations of discharge planners. Personally, discharge planners are overwhelmingly female (83%) and white (84%), with an average age of 36.

DISCHARGE PLANNING EFFECTIVENESS

How can discharge planning be made more effective? Specifically, what factors make discharge planning more effective in the eyes of discharge planners? To answer this question, we asked discharge planners "How well do you think the discharge planning process works in this hospital?" Table 2 shows the results of this analysis.

The analysis shows that the relationship between discharge planners and the rest of the hospital is more important than characteristics of the job in explaining effectiveness. Four factors are statistically significant in this analysis, the most important of them being the support and cooperation of the hospital administration. The administration must be willing to provide resources and overcome resistance to discharge planning for it to be effective.

The support of the administration also gives the discharge planners more influence in the hospital. Since planners have to coordinate so many resources and so many individuals with conflicting interests, they must have the power to win political battles in the hospital. Similarly, strong utilization review is also important, since it forces attention to be paid to discharge planning issues. The implementation of DRGs has had a similar effect.

The one job-related characteristic most closely related to effectiveness is the ability to change procedures easily. Discharge planners need flexibility to respond to changing needs, as well as a carefully conceived structure. If written discharge planning policy leads to rigid procedures, it is counterproductive.

Perhaps as interesting are those variables that are *not* significantly related to effective discharge planning. For example, the discharge planning model does not seem to relate systematically to effectiveness, nor does the reporting structure. More important is to increase the support and cooperation of the staff, whatever structure or model is used. Similarly, communication between the discharge

TABLE 2. VARIABLES RELATED TO DISCHARGE PLANNING EFFECTIVENESS.

Variable	Coefficient
Support and cooperation of hospital administration	.27
Ease of changing discharge planning procedures	.24
Influence of discharge planners in the hospital	.20
Importance of utilization review committee in the hospital	.11

N = 238   R-squared = .35

Note: The statistical method used is multiple regression, and the statistics reported are standardized regression coefficients (betas) for the regression equation in which discharge planning effectiveness is the dependent variable. Multiple regression shows the independent effect of each variable on the dependent variable. That is, each coefficient shows the effect of one variable on effectiveness when all other variables are taken into account. Each coefficient ranges between 0 (no relationship between effectiveness and the variable) and 1.0 (a perfect relationship between effectiveness and the variable). Only those variables that are significant at the .05 alpha level are included in the final equation.

planner and continuing care agencies outside the hospital is also not as important as relationships within the hospital. Even though they act as a bridge between acute and continuing care, discharge planners answer to the hospital staff, and the cooperation of that staff is more important than relationships with outside agencies.

Discharge planning is a facilitative role. In order to bring people together, the discharge planner must work well with a variety of people in the hospital. Having influence makes that interaction easier, as does the active support of the hospital administration. These factors should increase as prospective payment makes effective discharge planning more important to the viability of the hospital. This is the topic to which we next turn our attention.

DISCHARGE PLANNING AFTER PROSPECTIVE PAYMENT

The introduction of prospective payment for Medicare using diagnosis related groups (DRGs) in October 1983 began a new era for hospital discharge planning. A function that had been an unwanted stepchild in many hospitals suddenly became critical to the hospital's financial survival. Patients could only be released more quickly (thereby increasing the hospital's revenue) if discharge planning worked effectively. Although many authors have speculated on the effects (positive and negative) of DRGs on discharge planning, little empirical research has been done on this question. Our research provides a "before and after" picture of discharge planning by comparing discharge planning procedures before and after the introduction of DRGs.

Table 3 shows the major changes that have taken place within hospitals since the introduction of prospective payment. As many had predicted, discharge planning has received increased emphasis in the hospital under prospective payment. One of the anticipated changes was an increase in workload, and over half (56%) of the respondents reported such an increase. For those individuals, the caseload increased an average of 25 percent. However, this increase in work did not necessarily lead to an increase in staff. Only 21 percent said that the discharge planning staff had increased, and even then the addition was usually only one new staff member. It may well be that hospital staff patterns have not yet caught up with increased staffing needs, but more probably it means that discharge planners are simply expected to do more with the same resources.

Administratively, discharge planning has undergone some changes within the hospital. The use of interdisciplinary teams for discharge planning has increased, although only 11 percent report the creation of new full-time discharge planning units. One of the concerns about prospective payment was that since the hospital's fiscal well-being depended so heavily on timely patient discharge, hospital administration would exert more direct control by transferring discharge planning from social work or nursing to the administrator's office. This does not seem to be the case, since only 5 percent report that discharge planning has been transferred to this office.

TABLE 3. INTERNAL HOSPITAL CHANGES SINCE PROSPECTIVE PAYMENT.

| | Percentage | |
Characteristic	*YES*	*NO*
Discharge planning receives more emphasis in hospital	71	29
Increased workload (mean = 24%)	56	44
Increase staff for discharge planning (mode = 1)	21	79
Increased use of interdisciplinary teams	39	61
Creation of new full-time unit	11	89
Change in control to hospital administrator	5	95
Earlier access to patients	59	41
Increased preadmission screening	31	69
Earlier patient discharge (mean = 3 days)	71	29
Increased readmission rate	32	68

**TABLE 4.   EXTERNAL HOSPITAL CHANGES
SINCE PROSPECTIVE PAYMENT.**

Contact with continuing care agencies
   Increased   54%
   Remained the same   44%
   Decreased   2%
Measure posthospital adjustment of patients

	Time 1	Time 2
Yes	32%	15%
No	68%	85%

Increased interhospital competition
   Yes   45%
   No   55%
Forms of competition
   Increased marketing   46%
   Improved public services   23%
   Other (lower prices, 24-hour
      ER, regional referral service) 31%

The process of discharge planning has also changed. Discharge planners have earlier access to patients to screen for discharge problems, and one-third of all patients have preadmission discharge screening. Prospective payment is supposed to reduce the length of acute-care hospitalization, and 71 percent report that patients are discharged sooner, by an average of three days. One concern of critics of the new system is that quicker discharge will lead to increased readmissions, and about one-third report such an increase. However, it may be too early to reach a firm conclusion about the impact of DRGs on readmission rates.

Prospective payment has also changed relationships outside the hospital, as shown in Table 4. A majority of respondents (54%) report that contact with continuing care agencies (e.g., nursing homes, home health agencies) has increased. However, because of their increased workload, they are able to follow up on fewer patients than before DRGs, so that now only 15 percent report that they normally measure patients' posthospital adjustment.

Hospitals are also more aggressive in marketing their services in the competitive post-DRG marketplace, and almost half (45%) of respondents report an increase in competition between local hospitals. This generally takes the form of increased marketing or improved public relations. Since discharge planners are already involved in the community, some hospitals have looked to them to become more involved in public speaking for the hospital, although the percentage of those that do so is still small (24%).

Competition has forced hospitals to look for other ways to increase revenues, and for many this takes the form of "vertical integration," the process of incorporating into the hospital some services traditionally provided in the community. Table 5 shows the changes in hospital vertical integration that have taken place since DRGs. Hosital-based home care is the most popular of these, since some other

**TABLE 5.   HOSPITAL VERTICAL INTEGRATION SINCE
PROSPECTIVE PAYMENT.**

Since prospective payment, has hospital . . .	*Percentage Yes*
Begun patient home care training	30%
Begun hospital-based home care	21%
Begun day hospital	20%
Opened health related facility	17%
Begun sale of durable medical equipment	16%
Opened skilled nursing facility	9%
Contracted for nursing home beds	4%

TABLE 6. OUTCOME MEASURES SINCE PROSPECTIVE PAYMENT.

Discharge planning effectiveness
    (comparison between time 1 and time 2 answers)
    Less effective   33%
    No change   44%
    More effective   23%
Discharge planner satisfaction
    (comparison between time 1 and time 2 answers)
    Less satisfied   35%
    No change   40%
    More satisfied   25%

strategies (e.g., building a nursing home) involve much higher initial cost. This trend presents a dilemma for discharge planners. On the one hand, having a full range of services within the hospital organization makes discharge planning much simpler and is likely to enhance continuity of care for the patient. On the other hand, the discharge planner may be under pressure to use the hospital's services instead of reliable vendors in the community. Forcing the discharge planner to do so is illegal, but many discharge planners are fearful of the subtle pressure that might be exerted by hospital administration, especially if these services are making money for the hospital.

Finally, Table 6 shows the results of a comparison between times 1 and 2 on outcome variables. One-third of respondents felt that discharge planning was less effective since the implementation of prospective payment, while one-quarter saw an improvement. Approximately the same percentages feel less and more satisfied with their work as discharge planners.

While prospective payment using DRGs has greatly affected discharge planning by increasing its visibility and importance in the hospital, it has also increased the workload for those trying to cope with the changes. Many of the positive changes predicted for discharge planning after DRGs have yet to materialize. Perhaps a follow-up study in three or four years will show that such changes have taken place.

CONCLUSION

Hospital discharge planning is entering into a new era of increased responsibility, increased pressure, and increased power. Because of these changes, some of those presently working as discharge planners may not be in the same positions in five years. Increased visibility is a two-edged sword, since it both increases the influence of discharge planners and also invites the hospital administration to intervene in ways they previously have not. Discharge planners must take the initiative in defining their role, its possibilities, and its limitations. Hopefully, this report on research on discharge planning across the United States will help these professionals better understand the important role they fill in the health care system.

do not ignore the physician in discharge planning

Morris D. Kerstein
Ruth C. Baker
Maureen K. Maguire

The advent of prospective payment for health care is the most significant event since the enactment of Medicare and Medicaid legislation. There has never been greater need for emphasis on early discharge and posthospital care. The transfer of a patient from one health care setting to another frequently results in disruption of care rather than the required continuity. Chronic care or continuity of care does not have the charisma for most physicians that acute care does. The physician is further inhibited by the increasing numbers of regulatory and reimbursement policies. There may be an abundance of accessible, well-organized, community-based primary care systems for these populations, but the physician who works in the hospital environment has not until now felt a need to utilize these resources. Hospital financial stability requires appropriate early discharge and therefore requires that the physician be aware of those resources that facilitate the transfer of patients from the hospital to another multidisciplinary environment.

Hospitals vary widely in their approach to discharge planning; more than one-third (38%) have interdisciplinary teams consisting of nurses and social workers. Only 16 percent have full-time personnel with discharge planning as their sole responsibility. In many instances (more than 30%) there is a lone individual responsible for discharge planning. Despite the popularity of the team concept in health care, it is rarely implemented in U.S. hospitals. The discharge planner is often overburdened with other responsibilities, including counseling, patient care, administration, and utilization review. Hospital discharge planning has traditionally been the responsibility of two groups: nurses (26%) and social workers (52%). It appears that as discharge planning becomes a more important element in the hospital—and financial concerns will make it important—other health care professionals, such as physicians, accountants, and administrators, will become involved. The physician is an integral part of the discharge planning program and must be integrated into the discharge planning model used. Home health care or posthospital care is a basic component of health care delivery and includes a systematic coordination of patient needs with available resources. Comprehensive, coordinated service should be provided to meet patients' needs and facilitate their transfer from one level of care to another. A multidisciplinary, holistic approach should be used in planning with the patient, family, and significant others for their medical, therapeutic, rehabilitative, and psychosocial needs. The ultimate success of the plan depends on the involvement of the patient, family, and significant others in the decision-making process. We believe that the significant others include the physician.

On admission, each patient should be screened to determine his potential needs upon discharge. Criteria to be used to identify high-risk patients should be spelled out. There should be an increased awareness by all involved of the discharge planning process: the nurses on the floor as well as the social worker and administrative representative. The physician has to be made aware that the goal of admission is discharge, not permanent residence. There must be mechanisms established, such as rounds, conferences, or other methods of communicating information on changes in patients' status that might affect discharge. There should be a free flow of communication between the discharge planner (social worker or nurse), staff nurse, and primary physician. With this in mind, the patient and family must be involved in formulating and implementing a plan of discharge. If planning is done early, comprehensive patient information will be available to the receiving facility to use to evaluate the patient so as not to delay discharge. The physician must be made aware that this prompt planning program will not cause him to lose control or contact with his patient. Rather, a well-defined, organized method will have been established for continuity of care from admission to the hospital through discharge and final return to the physician's office for follow-up and evaluation.

Given the complex financial mechanisms that exist, files must be maintained on available community and state resources. Information on changes in internal and external regulations that affect health care must be readily available to the physician. The hospital should have professionals (nurse, administrator, or physician) who are responsible for maintaining the knowledge base. The physician will benefit from the flow of information about sources of funds. So long as the physician is kept aware of all options and regulations, he will respond in an appropriate fashion. As long as the system does not separate the physician from his patient, but rather facilitates the return of the patient to the primary physician in the outpatient setting, the physician will cooperate because it is in his best interest.

THE PHYSICIAN'S ROLE IN DISCHARGE PLANNING

The following series of events includes the steps involved in discharge planning as they affect the primary care physician or hospital-based physician. Patients in need of posthospital follow-up care should be identified on admission and evaluated by a health care professional with experience in discharge planning for the following high social risk factors: (1) age, (2) physical or mental handicaps, (3) noncompliance resulting in readmission, (4) abuse or neglect, (5) chemical dependency, (6) family crisis or conflict, (7) social isolation, (8) dependence, (9) insufficient financial resources, (10) inadequate housing, (11) need for transportation, and (12) transfer from another facility. It is evident that many elderly patients who are economically or socially deprived are at risk, and the problem is compounded by the limited number of external resources available for their discharge care. For this reason, these patients should be identified on admission, so that the physician can work with the discharge planner to arrange for postdischarge care.

A separate group identified as having high medical risks include patients with (1) chronic disease, (2) catastrophic illness, (3) high risk for exacerbation or difficult life-style readjustment, (4) communicable disease, (5) complex self-care requiring professional intervention, (6) inability to articulate realistic approaches to self-care; or (7) special needs. A patient with a catastrophic illness may need a chronic care center or specialized facilities. Because of the limited number of beds available in such settings, early identification of these patients will facilitate their transfer from acute-care hospitals to chronic care facilities. Another example would be a paraplegic who requires a great deal of equipment or assistance at home or the patient with chronic obstructive lung disease who needs various types of pulmonary support at home, including oxygen. Arrangement must be made before discharge, not only for the equipment but also for personnel to service it. Finally, even more important is a means by which the patient can seek outside help, whether it be the ability to dial 911 or an internal alarm system that will alert someone to seek emergency medical care.

The initial step in discharge planning is the systematic collection of subjective and objective data, so that an assessment of the patient's status can be obtained. This may require a patient interview or observation, evaluation of the medical records, input from hospital staff members, or other interviews.

Only through this mechanism can the patient's needs be determined. Among those with the most knowledge of the patient's needs and limitations is the primary care physician.

Planning reflects a systematic approach that meets the patient's individual needs. There are common disease processes but individual patients. A patient care conference may be needed, including all those involved in the patient's care, or discharge planning rounds. We emphasize that consultation with a physician is a requirement at this stage. If the physician is ignored, one can expect the patient to be referred back later for reassessment and reevaluation. Consultation with other health care professionals may be required, including the physical therapist, occupational therapist, and social worker, as long as the physician is involved and all data on the patient are integrated into a written discharge summary plan of care. The primary care to be given in the home or other setting should be specified, as should the patient's learning needs. Community resources must be investigated early in the planning process. Family support systems will help the patient adjust to the new setting, and the patient's adjustment is eased by the physician's knowledge of planning and his direct support of the planning mechanism and plans.

Everyone involved in the patient's care must be agreed that a continued approach to care is best. A discharge date should be projected and everyone should aim at that date, including in-house staff (nurses, physicians) and all related health care personnel. For practical reasons, the hospital administration needs a true assessment of the turnover of beds and bed utilization. Planning allows for this. Both the patient's and the family's knowledge of the disease process must be maximized by the date of discharge. When the patient arrives at home or in the chronic care facility, no one should have to make a frantic phone call back to the hospital to ask questions about the patient's medication status, family's knowledge, or future plans for rehabilitation.

If the patient is transferred to another acute-care facility, the social worker or nurse should have discussed the transfer with the patient's family and the receiving facility. The transfer date is then set by both receiving and sending services. At this point the physicians in both facilities will have been made aware of all problems so that no surprises will occur on either end. The transfer form (including all medical problems, discharge summary, medications, diet, activity, etc.) is transferred with the patient, but a copy of the form is sent ahead. A last-minute problem to be resolved is transportation for the patient, whether by wheelchair, litter, or with other mechanical support. The patient's success in rehabilitation is clearly a product of all those contributing to his transfer. The social worker and nurse, working with the discharge planner and finally the primary care physician, should confirm the patient's individual and family's long-term needs. If the level of care required is clearly specified, there should be little chance for lack of continuity of care that can disrupt the patient's rehabilitation. Among the many problems that seem to occur is lack of completion of referral forms, discharge planning forms, and other medical information. If the physician is given sufficient advance notice, these forms can be completed with a minimum of anxiety and aggravation.

Follow-up Evaluation

The physician's role in follow-up evaluation is to confirm that the process is working and the desired goals are attained. Throughout the system means of communication should be established with clinicians, the primary physician, clinic nurses, social workers, patient, and family.

DISCHARGE PLANNING ROUNDS

The physician can most easily play an integral role in discharge planning through the mechanism of discharge planning rounds. The easiest system entails combined patient care rounds one day a week in the company of the staff nurse, social worker, discharge planning nurse, and utilization review nurse, with the staff physician or resident presenting each case to the group. The case should be presented in the same context as it normally would be: patient's name, age, diagnosis, date of admission, and chief complaint. Also, the patient's history and physical status and the results of diagnostic and therapeutic procedures should be mentioned. The patient's prognosis should be clearly described, including functional limitations, mental status, and bodily function, or performance of the activities of daily living. The physician should then state the projected date of discharge. Questions can be generated by the group, available support systems, living arrangements, family response to illness, social and economic needs, and whether home health care services or long term care facilities will be required. In context, the physician can easily make the appropriate assessment or seek assistance from others present. Discharge planning rounds thus allow the physician to identify the discharge plan and date, status of the patient, the family's knowledge of his condition, and the ability of the patient and family to provide care. There should be a discharge care note made in the chart so that everyone will be aware of the current status of discharge planning.

It is clear that the physician plays an integral role in identifying the patient's capabilities, both physical and mental. The physician should be available for consultation with the discharge planner, staff nurse, and receiving facility. The secret to success, of course, is communication and coordination among all members of the multidisciplinary health care team. Given the necessary information, the physician will play an integral role in discharge planning for the patient.

Discharge planning for continuity of care will increase in importance as regulatory and financial constraints continue to emphasize cost control. The physician's participation in discharge planning must benefit both the institution and the physician. It is clear that discharge planning will become a higher priority in every hospital than it has been in the past. Discharge planning units will be given more staff, resources, and influence; but the hospital's administration may directly control the discharge planning process. All professional groups must become actively involved in discharge planning and, subsequently, in the political activities carried out to regulate discharge planning.

notes

CHAPTER 1

1. Clement Bezold, "Medical Megatrends Reshaping Delivery and Evaluation of Care," *Modern Health-care* (July 1984): 165

2. "PSROs Turn Pro," *The AMPRA Review* (July–August 1984): 1.

3. Susan Lee, "Enough Is Enough," *Forbes*, September 10, 1984, p. 109.

4. *Introduction to Discharge Planning for Hospitals* (Chicago: American Hospital Association), 1.

5. *Turf Problem Task Force Report* (Washington, D.C.: American Association for Continuity of Care), 1.

6. B. Joan Newcomb, "Discharge Planning in the Progressive Era," *Discharge Planning Update* (Summer 1982): 10–11.

7. "Introduction," *Discharge Planning Fact Pack* (Philadelphia: University of Pennsylvania National Health Care Management Center), 1–5.

8. Faith Jackson Crittenden, *Discharge Planning for Health Care Facilities* (Bowie, Md.: Brady Communications), 5.

CHAPTER 2

1. American Nurses' Association, *Continuity of Care and Discharge Planning Programs* (New York: The Association, 1975), 3.

2. *Ibid.*

3. *Ibid.*, 2.

4. U.S. National Advisory Commission on Health Facilities, *A Report to the President* (Washington, D.C.: U.S. Government Printing Office, 1968), 1–54.

5. *Ibid.*

6. American Hospital Association, *Quality Assurance Program* (Chicago: The Association, 1972).

7. American Hospital Association, *Statement on a Patient's Bill of Rights.* (Chicago: The Association, 1972).

8. Brookdale Hospital Medical Center, "Discharge Planning Protocol," Brooklyn, New York, June, 1975.

CHAPTER 3

1. Paul L. Grimaldi, "Public Law 97–248: The Implication of Prospective Payment Schedules," *Nursing Management* (February 1983): 25.

2. American Hospital Association, *Special Report 3: Medicare Prospective Pricing* (Chicago: The Association, 1983).

3. John Feather and Linda Nichols, "Profile: A National Perspective on Discharge Planning," *The Next Step* (September 1984): 2–3.

4. American Hospital Association, *Special Report 7: Medicare Payment—Cost-per-Case Management* (Chicago: The Association, 1983).

5. American Hospital Association, *Special Report 6: Medicare Prospective Pricing—Summary of Regulations* (Chicago: The Association, 1983).

6. JCAH, *Accreditation Manual for Hospitals* (Chicago: The Commission, 1984), 114.

7. *Ibid.*, 193.

8. American Hospital Association, *Guidelines for Discharge Planning* (Chicago: The Association, 1984).

9. American Nurses' Association, *Continuity of Care and Discharge Planning Programs* (New York: The Association, 1975), 6.

10. U.S. Department of Health, Education, and Welfare, *Professional Standards Review Organizations Manual* (Washington D.C.: U.S. Government Printing Office, 1974).

CHAPTER 4

1. Joan Clemons, "Basic Discharge Planning: A Mini-Course," *The Coordinator* (May 1984): 36. Reprinted by permission.
2. James McNamara and Harold Smith, *Discharge Planning Proposal*, University Hospital, University of Utah Medical Center, Salt Lake City, 1984 (unpublished).
3. Montefiore Hospital Home Care Department, *Home Health Services: Selected Papers*, Pittsburgh, 1970, p. 25.
4. Commission on Professional and Hospital Activities, *Length of Stay by Diagnosis* (Ann Arbor, Mich.: The Commission, 1983).
5. Montefiore Hospital Home Care Department, *op. cit.*, 25–26.
6. Carol W. Soskis, "Discharge Planning for the Emergency Department Social Worker," *Discharge Planning Update* (Summer 1983): 8–9.
7. U.S. Department of Health, Education, and Welfare, Health Services and Mental Health Administration, *EMCRO Notebook*, Pub. No. (HSM) 73-3017 (Washington, D.C.: U.S. Government Printing Office, 1973), 132–138.
8. David Simpson, "Patient Discharge Planning," *Journal of the Albert Einstein Medical Center* 17 (Autumn 1969).

CHAPTER 5

1. American Hospital Association, *Introduction to Discharge Planning for Hospitals* (Chicago: The Association, 1983).
2. Claudia J. Coulton, "Discharge Planning and Decision Making," *Health and Social Work*, November 1982.
3. Thomas Holland, "Ethical Issues Facing Discharge Planners," *Discharge Planning Update*, Winter 1984.
4. American Hospital Association, *op. cit.*

CHAPTER 6

1. Paul Kleyman, "American Association of Continuity of Care Conference Report," *The Coordinator* (December 1984): 43.
2. "Establishing a Discharge Planning Model," document prepared for the New York City Health and Hospitals Corporation, June 1978.
3. Long Island College Hospital, Brooklyn, New York, "Discharge Planning Model," *Discharge Planning Update* (Summer 1983): 25.
4. *Ibid.*, 25–28.
5. Brookdale Hospital Medical Center, "Discharge Planning Protocol," Brooklyn, New York, 1975.

CHAPTER 7

1. American Hospital Association, *Guidlines for Discharge Planning* (Chicago: The Association, 1984), 2.
2. Cynthia W. Sanborn and Mary Blount, "Standard Plans for Care and Discharge," *American Journal of Nursing* (November 1984): 1394–1396.
3. U.S. Department of Health, Education, and Welfare, Health Services and Mental Health Administration, *Continuity of Care Through Discharge Planning* (Washington, D.C.: U.S. Government Printing Office).
4. Thomas Antone, *Discharge Planning* (Washington, D.C.: U.S. Government Printing Office), 1.
5. Silver Cross Hospital, Joliet, Illinois, "Discharge Planning Model," *Discharge Planning Update* (Spring 1982): 21–29.
6. Long Island College Hospital, Brooklyn, New York, "Discharge Planning Model," *Discharge Planning Update* (September 1983): 24–32.
7. Oakwood Hospital, Dearborn, Michigan, "Discharge Planning Model," *Discharge Planning Update* (Summer 1982): 26–34.

CHAPTER 11

1. I. M. Cannon, *On the Social Frontier of Medicine: Pioneering in Medical Social Service* (Cambridge, Mass.: Harvard University Press, 1952), 14.
2. Sherry L. Shamansky, Janice Carol Boase, and Beverly M. Horn, "Discharge Planning: Yesterday, Today, and Tomorrow," *Home Health Care Nurse* (May–June 1984): 14–21.

3. American Hospital Association, *A Patient's Bill of Rights* (Chicago: The Association, 1972).

4. G. Hushower, D. Gamberg, and N. Smith, "The Nursing Process in Discharge Planning," *Supervisor Nurse* (September 1978): 55–58; R. W. Weinback, "Dispelling the Myths of Discharge Planning," *Southern Hospital* (1976): 17.

5. Cynthia M. Runner-Heidt, "Where Does the Hospital Discharge Planner Go From Here?" *Home Health Care Nurse* (July–August 1984): 30–35.

6. Winifred Livingood, Carolyn Smith, and Sandra Hallstead, "The Impact of DRGs on Home Health Care," *Home Health Care Nurse* (September–October 1983): 29.

CHAPTER 12

1. R. C. Edwards, "Professionals in 'Alliance' Achieve More Effective Discharge Planning," *Journal of Gerontological Nursing* 5 (1978): 34–39; J. C. Simmons, "A Reporting System for Hospital Social Services Departments," *Health and Social Work* 3 (1978): 100–112; M. Brown and M. Kiss, "Discharge Planning: A Quality Assurance Program in a Cancer Research Hospital," *Cancer Nursing* 3 (1980): 138–144; R. M. Spano and S. M. Lund, "Accountability, Evaluation, and Quality Assurance in a Hospital Social Service Department," *Quality Review Bulletin* 6 (1980): 14–19.

2. P. A. Reichelt and J. Newcomb, "Organizational Factors in Discharge Planning," *Journal of Nursing Administration* 10 (1980): 36–42; Greater New York Hospital Association, *Hospital Discharge Planning—A Confusing Route to a Simple Goal* (New York: The Association, 1980); *Study of Hospital Discharges for Patients 65 and Over* (New York: The Association, 1980); *Study of Patients Between the Ages of 18 and 64 Discharged from Two Voluntary Acute Care Hospitals in New York City* (New York: The Association, 1981); P. Livingston, "After Service Needs Assessment for Older Persons with a Disability," New York University reprint, 1981.

3. C. Helbing, *Ten Years of Short-Stay Hospital Utilization and Costs Under Medicare: 1967–1976* (Washington, D.C.: Health Care Financing Administration, 1980); S. Kretz, "Changing Patterns of Entry into Home Health Services," Office of Service Delivery Assessment, U.S. Department of Health and Human Services, 1981; C. P. Monier, M. M. Makowiecki, and M. R. Yessian, "Medicare Home Health Services: A Service Delivery Assessment," Office of Service Delivery Assessment, U.S. Department of Health and Human Services, 1981; J. Berke, "The Spread of Discharge Management: New Definitions, New Careers, New Power," *The Coordinator* (October 1984): 16–26.

bibliography

Adams, J. "Alternate Forms of Care Benefit Young and Old." *Hospitals* 54 (May 16, 1980): 91–94.

Alfano, G. J. "The Nurse's Impact on Effective Discharge Planning." *Discharge Planning Update* 3 (Summer 1982): 4–6.

American Academy of Pediatrics Committee on Fetus and Newborn. "Criteria for Early Infant Discharge and Follow-up Evaluation." *Pediatrics* 65, no. 3 (1980): 651.

American Hospital Association. *Guidelines: Discharge Planning.* Chicago: The Association, 1984.

———. *Introduction to Discharge Planning for Hospitals.* Chicago: The Association, 1983.

———. *A Patient's Bill of Rights.* Chicago: The Association, 1972.

———. *Quality Assurance Program.* Chicago: The Association, 1972.

———. *Special Report 3: Medicare Prospective Pricing.* Chicago: The Association, 1983.

———. *Special Report 6: Medicare Prospective Pricing—Summary of Regulations.* Chicago: The Association, 1983.

———. *Special Report 7: Medicare payment—Cost-per-Case Management.* Chicago: The Association, 1983.

American Nurses' Association. *Community Health Nursing Practice Standards.* New York: The Association, 1973.

———. *Continuity of Care and Discharge Planning Programs in Institutions and Community Agencies.* New York: The Association, 1975.

———. *Nursing and Long Term Care: Toward Quality Care for the Aging.* New York: The Association, 1975.

Anderson, Cynthia A. "Home or Nursing Home? Let the Elderly Patient Decide." *American Journal of Nursing* 79 (August 1979): 1449–1450.

———. "Making the Right Moves in Discharge Planning: Home or Nursing Home? Let the Elderly Patient Decide." *American Journal of Nursing* 79 (August 1979): 1448–1449.

Armitage, S. K. "Negotiating the Discharge of Medical Patients." *Journal of Advanced Nursing* 6 (September 1981): 8–11.

Aroskar, Mila A. "Ethical Issues in Community Health Nursing." *Nursing Clinics of North America* 14 (March 1979): 35–44.

Austin, S. E. J. "Family-Centered Discharge Planning Classes: Postpartum Instruction." *MCN* 5 (March–April 1980): 96–97.

Avery, M. D., et al. "An Early Postpartum Hospital Discharge Program: Implementation and Evaluation." JOGN 11 (July–August 1982): 233–235.

Bachman, C., and K. Preston. "Effective Rehabilitation: Reintegration into the Community." *Rehabilitation Nursing* 9 (January–February 1984): 14–16.

Barry, Kathryn. "A Discharge Planning Protocol Conceptualized by a Clinical Nurse Specialist." *Rehabilitation Nursing* 8 (September–October 1983): 27–30.

Batey, S. R., et al. "Using a Resource Group to Coordinate Services in Discharge Planning." *Hospital and Community Psychiatry* 31 (1980): 417–418.

Beatty, Sally. *Continuity of Care, the Hospital, and the Community.* New York: Grune & Stratton, 1980.

Bennett, C. "Testing the Value of Written Information for Patients and Families in Discharge Planning." *Social Work in Health Care* 9 (Spring 1984): 95–100.

Berns, J. "Inpatient Discharge Planning." *Journal of the Indiana State Medical Association* 73 (June 1980): 366–368.

Bezold, Clement. "Medical Megatrends Reshaping Delivery and Evaluation of Care." *Modern Healthcare* (July 1984): 165.

Brando, Alvin B. "An Overview of Discharge Planning." *N.I.M.H. Information Bulletin* (January 1981).

Britton, C., et al. "Innovative Discharge Planning—Try It; The Result May Surprise You." *Nursing 80* (October 1980): 44–49.

Brody, S. J., and C. Mascrocchi. "Data for Long Term Care Planning." *American Journal of Public Health* 70 (November 1980): 1194–1198.

Bromfield, S. "Involving Staff in Discharge Planning." *Supervisor Nurse* 10 (May 1979): 35–38.

Brookdale Hospital Medical Center. *Discharge Planning Protocol.* Brooklyn, N.Y.: Brookdale Hospital Medical Center, 1975.

———. *Brook Lodge Symposium—Discharge Planning to Home Care.* Upjohn Health Care Services, May 1982.

Burkey, S. "An Audit Outcome: Home-Going Instructions." *Supervisor Nurse* 10 (May 1979): 36.

Cagan, J., and P. Meier. "A Discharge Planning Tool for Use With Families of High-Risk Infants." JOGN 8 (May–June 1979): 146–148.

Cahill, T. F. "Prospective Reimbursement: Its Effects on Discharge Planning Services." *Discharge Planning Update* 3 (Fall 1982): 14–16.

Caldwell, J. "Whatever Happened to Intermediate Care?" *Journal of Long Term Care Administration* 9 (Winter 1981): 34–42.

Campbell, A. J. M., and A. J. Mehta. "Outpatient Rehabilitation Center Keeps Many Elderly Living at Home." *Hospitals* 55 (June 16, 1981): 101–102, 105.

Cannon, I. M. *On the Social Frontier of Medicine: Pioneering in Medical Social Service.* Cambridge, Mass.: Harvard University Press, 1952.

Chisolm, Mary M. "Promises and Pitfalls of Discharge Planning." *Nursing Management* 14 (November 1983): 26–29.

Christy, N. W., and C. Frasca. "The Benefits of Hospital-Sponsored Home Care Programs." *Journal of Nursing Administration* 13 (December 1983): 7–10.

Clemons, Joan. "Basic Discharge Planning: A Mini-Course." *The Coordinator* 2 (May 1984): 34–38.

Cohen, Elias. "Legal Consequences of Continuity of Care Decisions." *The Coordinator* 2 (May 1984): 10–11.

Coleman, John. "DRGs and the Growth of Home Health." *Economic Issues* 2 (November–December 1984).

"Combined Functions Ensure Patients' Continuity of Care." *Hospital Progress* 64 (March 1983): 26–30.

Commission on Professional and Hospital Activities. *Length of Stay by Diagnosis.* Ann Arbor, Mich.: The Commission, 1983.

Conger, Shirley A., and L. F. Snider. "The Priority Component of Discharge Planning." *The Coordinator* 1 (December 1983): 16–20.

Connally, M. L. "Organize Your Work Day for More Effective Discharge Planning." *Nursing 81* (July 1981): 44–47.

Coon, M., T. LaMotte, and M. J. Stanton. "Continuity of Care Aim of Program." *Hospitals* 55 (September 16, 1981): 81, 84.

Cooper, J. "Helping the Elderly to Leave the Hospital: Patient Thinking." *Nursing Mirror* 153 (August 12, 1983): 26–27.

Copp, L. A. *Responding to Stress: Community Mental Health in the 80's.* New York: National League for Nursing, 1981.

Coulton, C. J., et al. "Discharge Planning and Decision Making." *Health and Social Work* 7 (November 1982): 253–261.

Coulton, Claudia. "Implementing Quality Assurance." *The Coordinator* 1 (January 1983): 18–19.

———. Counseling the Patient and Family Unit Regarding the Home Care Options in Discharge Planning." *The Baton* (Upjohn Health Care, Kalamazoo, Michigan) 1 (January 1984).

Crittenden, Faith Jackson. *Discharge Planning for Health Care Facilities.* Bowie, Maryland: Brady, 1983.

Delaney, M. C., and J. Trachtenberg. "Discharge Planning: A Quality Assurance Program in a Cancer Research Hospital." *Cancer Nursing* 3 (April 1980): 138–144.

Demilo, K. L., and P. M. Campbell. "Improving Hospital Discharge Data: Lessons from the National Hospital Discharge Survey." *Medical Care* 19 (October 1981): 1030–1040.

DeYoung, M. "Care of the Acutely Ill Older Adult: Planning for Discharge." *Geriatric Nursing* 3 (November–December 1982): 396–399.

———. "Discharge Planning Improves Aftercare for Elderly." *Hospital Progress* 64 (January 1983): 22–24.

———. "Discharge Planning Model—Long Island College Hospital, Brooklyn, N.Y." *Discharge Planning Update* 4 (Summer 1983): 25–28.

———. "Discharge Planning Model—Silver Cross Hospital, Joliet, IL." *Discharge Planning Update* (Spring 1982).

———. "Discharge Planning Models: Models Revisited." *Discharge Planning Update* 4 (Fall 1983): 30–34.

Dunkee, R., et al. "Factors Affecting Post-Hospital Care Planning of Elderly Patients in an Acute Care Setting." *Journal of Gerontological Social Work* 4 (Spring–Summer 1982): 95–101.

Dunlop, B. D. "Expanded Home-Based Care for the Impaired Elderly: Solution or Pipe Dream?" *American Journal of Public Health* 90 (May 1980): 514–518.

———. *Establishing a Discharge Planning Model.* New York: Prepared for the New York City Health and Hospitals Corporation, June, 1978.

Feather, John, and Linda Nichols. "Hospital Discharge Planning: The Other Side of Continuity of Care." *Caring* (October 1984): 37–38.

Feather, John, and Linda Nichols. "Profile: A National Perspective on Hospital Discharge Planning." *The Next Step* (The Glass Rock Home Health Care Newsletter for Discharge Planning) 1 (September 1984).

Gikow, F. F. "A Decision Model—How to Determine Appropriate Community Services for the Elderly." *Nursing & Health Care* 2 (June 1981): 322–326.

Glover, J. C. "Reducing Discharge Planning Paperwork with Pocket-Size Discharge Planning Record." *Nursing 81* (December 1981): 50–51.

Golightly, C., et al. "Planning to Meet the Needs of the Hospitalized Elderly." *The Journal of Nursing Administration* 4 (May 1984): 29–38.

Grimaldi, Paul L. "Public Law 97–248: The Implications of Prospective Payment Schedules." *Nursing Management* 14 (February 1983): 25–27.

Habeeb, M. C. "Information Management in Discharge Planning: Future Directions." *Discharge Planning Update* 3 (Spring 1982): 5–7.

Habeeb, M. C., and Frank E. McLaughlin. "Making the Right Moves in Discharge Planning Including the Hospital Staff Nurse." *American Journal of Nursing* 79 (August 1979): 1443–1445.

Harvey, B. "Your Patient's Discharge Plan: Does It Include Home Care Referral." *Nursing 81* (July 1981): 48–51.

Holland, Thomas. "Ethical Issues Facing Discharge Planners." *Discharge Planning Update* (Winter 1984).

Huey, R. "Discharge Planning: Good Planning Means Fewer Hospitalizations for the Chronically Ill." *Nursing 81* (May 1981): 44–50.

Hushower, G., D. Gamberg, and N. Smith. "The Nursing Process in Discharge Planning." *Supervisor Nurse* 9 (September 1978): 55–58.

Illinois Council of Home Health Services. *Home Health Care: A Consumer Guide.* Evanston: The Council.

Jessee, W. F., and B. J. Doyle. "Discharge Planning: Using Audits to Identify Areas that Need Improvement." *Quality Review Bulletin* (Spring 1982): 62–65.

Johnson, J., et al. "Planning Patients' Discharge." *Supervisor Nurse* 12 (February 1981): 44.

Joint Commission on Accreditation of Hospitals. *Accreditation Manual for Hospitals.* Chicago: The Commission, 1984.

Kane, R. "Discharge Planning: An Undischarged Responsibility?" *Health Social Work* 5 (February 1980): 2–3.

Kleyman, Paul. "American Association for Continuity of Care: Turf Issues and Discharge Planning After DRG's Explored at AACC's Third Annual Conference." *The Coordinator* 2 (December 1984): 43.

Knight, Marilyn. "A Nursing Home: Sometimes the Only Answer." *HomeLife* (January 1984): 43–45.

Kozak, L. J., et al. "The Status of Hospital Discharge Data in Six Countries." *Vital Health Statistics* 12 (March 1980): 1–77.

Kulys, Regina. "Future Crisis and the Very Old: Implications for Discharge Planning: Implications for Social Workers." *Health and Social Work* 8 (Summer 1983): 182–195.

Kurland, C. "The Medical Day Care Program in New Jersey." *Home Health Care Services Quarterly* 3 (Summer 1982): 45–61.

LaMontagne, M., and M. McKeehan. "Profile of a Continuing Care Program Emphasizing Discharge Planning." *The Journal of Nursing Administration* 5 (October 1975): 22–25.

Lamont, Campbell T., Susan Sampson, Ruth Matthias, and Robert Kane. "The Outcome of Hospitalization for Acute Illness in the Elderly." *Journal of the American Geriatric Society* 31 (May 1983): 282–287.

Lesse, J. S., and B. J. Reilly. "Assessing the Outcomes of a Home Nursing Program: Previously Hospitalized Versus Nonhospitalized Patients." *Journal of Advanced Nursing* 5 (November 1980): 561–572.

Levey, S. "Study Pinpoints Consequences of Poor D/P Interview." *Hospital Peer Review* (February 1981).

Lindenberg, R. E., et al. "Planning for Posthospital Care: A Follow-up Study." *Health Social Work* 5 (February 1980): 45–50.

Livingood, Winifred S., Caroly Smith, and Sandra Hallstead. "The Impact of DRGs on Home Health Care." *Home Health Care Nurse* 1 (September–October 1983): 29.

Lynnwood, W. A. "I'd Rather Be Home: A Practical Guide for Individual Families and Professionals." Appro Printing, 1983.

McCann, B. A. "Hospice Care: A Challenge and an Opportunity for Discharge Planners." *Discharge Planning Update* 4 (Fall 1983): 6–10.

McCarthy, S. A. "Discharge Planning in a Primary Nursing System." *Discharge Planning Update* 4 (Fall 1983): 10–14.

McKeehan, D. "Nursing Diagnosis in a Discharge Planning Program." *Nursing Clinics of North America* 14 (1979): 517–524.

McKeehan, Kathleen. "The Role of the Client in Discharge Planning Teamwork." *Discharge Planning Update* (Winter 1982).

McKeehan, K. M. (ed). *Continuing Care: A Multidisciplinary Approach to Discharge Planning.* St. Louis: C. V. Mosby, 1981.

McNamara, James, and Harold Smith. "Discharge Planning Proposal." Salt Lake City: University Hospital, University of Utah Medical Center, 1984. Unpublished.

McPhee, S. J., et al. "Influence of a 'Discharge Interview' on Patient Knowledge, Compliance, and Functional Status After Hospitalization." *Medical Care* 21 (August 1983): 755–767.

Martin, A. "How to Help When a Patient Goes Home to Die." *Nursing Life* 1 (September–October 1981): 66–71.

Martin, N., et al. (eds). *Comprehensive Rehabilitation Nursing.* New York: McGraw-Hill, 1981.

Mezzonotte, E. Jane. "A Checklist for Better Discharge Planning." *Nursing 80* (November 1980): 64.

Montefiore Hospital, Home Care Department. *Home Health Services—Selected Papers.* Pittsburgh: Montefiore Hospital, 1970.

Moore, M. F. "Head Nurses Become Effective Managers in Discharge Planning Process." *Discharge Planning Update* 4 (Fall 1983): 15–17.

Morales, M., et al. "The Dynamics of a Geriatric Day Hospital." *Age and Aging* 13 (January 1984): 34–41.

Moxley, J. H., and P. C. Roeder. "New Opportunities for Out-Of-Hospital Health Services." *New England Journal of Medicine* 310 (January 19, 1984): 193–197.

Mullaney, J. W., et al. "Legal Problems and Principles in Discharge Planning: Implications for Social Work." *Social Work in Health Care* 9 (Fall 1983): 53–62.

Mundinger, Mary O'Neil. *Home Care Controversy.* Rockville, Md.: Aspen Systems Corporation, 1983.

Mundy, Rodrigo, and Betty Mesick. "Hospitalization of the Elderly for Acute Illness." *Journal of the American Geriatric Society* 27 (September 1979): 415–417.

Murray, Louisa M. "Summary of Invitational Conference, South Hills Health System Home Health Agency." Unpublished Report Prepared for Baptist Hospital of Miami. June 1983.

Newcomb, Joan B. "Discharge Planning in the Progressive Era." *Discharge Planning Update* 3 (Summer 1982): 10–11.

Nichols, Linda, and John Feather. "Discharge Planning." *Homecare* (April 1984): 80–84.

———. "Factors Influencing Discharge Planning Effectiveness and Job Satisfaction." *The Coordinator* 2 (May 1984): 43–45.

———. *Nursing and Long Term Care: Toward Quality Care for the Aging.* New York: American Nurses' Association, 1975.

Oakwood Hospital, Dearborn, Mich. "Discharge Planning Model." *Discharge Planning Update* (Summer 1982).

O'Brien, C. "Elderly Day Health Care." *American Health Care Association Journal* 5 (September 1979): 3–6.

O'Neil, E. A. "Exclusive Referral Agreements for Home Care: Affiliation Between the Hospital and a Community Home Health Agency." *Nursing Economics* 2 (September–October 1984): 326–328, 364.

Palmer, E., et al. "Discharge Planning: Effect on Length of Hospital Stay." *Archives of Physical Medicine and Rehabilitation* 64 (February 1983): 57–60.

Podalsky, Rose, and James H. Mason. "Geriatric Discharge Planning and Follow-up." *Illinois Medical Journal* 157 (May 1980): 291–292.

Prichard, M. A. "Communications: A Concept of Continuing Care." *Nursing Times* 76 (January 24, 1980): 169–172.

Raitt, J., et al. "Manual Helps Formalize Discharge Planning Services." *Dimensions in Health Service* 61 (April 1984): 29–30.

Rasmusen, Linda. "A Screening Tool Promotes Early Discharge Planning." *Nursing Management* 15 (May 1984): 39–40, 42–43.

Ratcliff, Basom. *Leaving the Hospital: Discharge Planning for Total Patient Care.* Springfield, Ill.: Charles C. Thomas, 1981.

Reichelt, Paul A., et al. "Organizational Factors in Discharge Planning: Four Models." *Journal of Nursing Administration* 10 (December 1980): 36–42.

Reiff, Theodore R. "When a Patient Is Admitted to a Nursing Home." *Geriatrics* 35 (July 1980): 87–94.

Reilly, M. "Let's Set the Record Straight: Preparing the Discharge Summary and the Patient's Instruction Sheet." *Nursing 79* (January 1979): 55–60.

Romano, C. A. "A Computerized Approach to Discharge Care Planning." *Nursing Outlook* 32 (January–February 1984): 23–25.

Roselle, Sue, and Frank D'Amico. "The Effects of Home Respiratory Therapy on Hospital Readmission Rates of Patients with Chronic Obstructive Pulmonary Disease." *Respiratory Care* 27 (October 1982): 1194–1199.

Rosen, Rosalind P. "Alzheimer's Disease: A Guide for the Discharge Planner." *The Coordinator* 2 (January 1984): 19–21.

Rosenthal, J. M., and D. B. Miller. "Providers Have Failed to Work for Continuity." *Hospitals* 53 (May 16, 1979): 79–83.

Rossen, S. "Adapting Discharge Planning to Prospective Pricing." *Hospitals* 58 (March 1, 1984): 71, 75, 79.

Rowland, H. S., and B. L. Rowland. "Patient Education and Patient Discharge." In *Nursing Administration Handbook.* Germantown, Md.: Aspen Systems Corporation, 1980.

Runner-Heidt, Cynthia M. "Where Does the Hospital Discharge Planner Go from Here?" *Home Health Care Nurse* 2 (July–August 1984): 30–31, 34–35.

Rutkin-Pearlman, Irene. "Discharge Planning: The Team Is Behind You!" *Nursing Management* 15 (May 1984): 36–38.

Sanborn, Cynthia W., and Mary Blount. "Standard Plans for Care and Discharge." *American Journal of Nursing* 84 (November 1984): 1394–1396.

Scupholme, A. "Postpartum Early Discharge: An Inner City Experience." *Journal of Nurse Midwifery* 26 (November–December 1981): 19–22.

Shaffer, Frank. "Nursing Power in the DRG World." *Nursing Management* 15 (June 1984): 28–30.

Shamansky, S. L., et al. "Discharge Planning: Yesterday, Today and Tomorrow." *Home Healthcare Nurse* 2 (May–June 1984): 14–17, 20–21.

Shine, M. S. "Discharge Planning for the Elderly in Acute Care Setting." *Nursing Clinics of North America* 18 (June 1983): 403–410.

Shulman, L., and L. Tuzman. "Discharge Planning: A Social Work Perspective." *Quality Review Bulletin* 6 (October 1980): 3–8.

Simmons, John C. "Discharge Management: Its Future." *Home Health Care Update* (Fall 1982).

Simpson, David. "Patient Discharge Planning." *Journal of the Albert Einstein Medical Center* (Autumn 1969).

Smith, D. M., et al. "Hospital Discharge Data Used as Feedback in Planning Research and Education for Primary Care." *Public Health Reports* 98 (September–October 1983): 1462–1467.

Smith, J. A., J. Buckalew, and S. M. Rosales. "Making the Right Moves in Discharge Planning: Coordinating a Workable System." *American Journal of Nursing* 79 (August 1979): 1439–1440.

Soskis, Carol W. "Discharge Planning for the Emergency Department Social Worker." *Discharge Planning Update* 4 (Summer 1983): 8–11.

Steffl, Bernita M., and I. Eide. *Discharge Planning Handbook*. Thorofare, N.J.: Charles B. Slack, 1978.

Stone, M. "Making the Right Moves in Discharge Planning: Discharge Planning Guide." *American Journal of Nursing* 79 (August 1979): 1446–1447.

———. "Strategies Given for Discharge Planning Activities." *Hospitals* 58 (July 16, 1984): 72, 76.

Sullivan, J. "Continuity of Care Between Hospital and Home." *Nursing Administration Quarterly* 6 (Fall 1981): 19–22.

Supiand, K. P., and N. L. Peacock. "Discharge Planning for Residents of a Long Term Care Facility." *Quality Review Bulletin* 7 (October 1981): 17–25.

Tebbitt, B. V. "What's Happening in Continuity of Care?" *Supervisor Nurse* 12 (March 1981): 22.

Tessler, R., and J. H. Mason. "Continuity of Care in the Delivery of Mental Health Services." *American Journal of Psychiatry* 136 (October 1979): 1297–1301.

Thomas, Antone. *Discharge Planning*. Washington, D.C.: U.S. Government Printing Office.

Thomasma, David C. "Limitations of the Autonomy Model for the Doctor–Patient Relationship." *The Pharos* 46 (Spring 1983): 2–5.

United States Department of Health, Education and Welfare. *Professional Standards Review Organizational Manual*. Washington, D.C.: U.S. Government Printing Office, 1974.

United States Department of Health, Education and Welfare, Health Services and Mental Health Administration. *EMCRO Notebook* (Pub. No. HSM 73-3017). Washington, D.C.: U.S. Government Printing Office, 1973.

United States National Advisory Commission of Health Facilities. *A Report to the President, December, 1968*.

Washington, D.C.: U.S. Government Printing Office, 1968.

Urosevich, Patti. "How Nurses are Learning to Live with DRGs." *Nursing Life* 4 (March–April 1984): 64–65.

Vlack, J. E., and M. G. Connolly. "Making the Right Moves in Discharge Planning: When a Nursing Home is the Best Choice." *American Journal of Nursing* 79 (August 1979): 1450–1451.

Walczak, Regina. "The New JCAH Quality Assurance Standards—Their Impact on Continuity of Care." *The Coordinator* 1 (January 1983): 16–21.

Waters, Elva Jane. *How to Do Patient Discharge Planning*. Miami: Author, 1980.

Wells, James B. "Interfacing Hospitals and Home Health Care Providers." *Caring* (July 1984): 35–36.

Wells, M. "Discharge Planning: Closing the Gaps in Continuity of Care." *Nursing 83* (November 1983): 45.

Wilson-Haas, Sheila A. "Sorting Out Nursing Productivity." *Nursing Management* 15 (April 1984): 37–40.

Worshow, Gregg A. "Hospital Care for Elderly Patients." *Duke University Center Reports on Advances in Research* 7 (December 1983): 1–7.

Wright, H., and A. Lacot. "From Hospital to Nursing Home: Evaluation Plan Helps Bridge the Gap Between Acute and Long Term Care Concerns." *Quality Review Bulletin* 6 (August 1980): 7–10.

Youssef, F. A. "Compliance with Therapeutic Regimens: A Follow-up Study for Patients with Affective Disorders." *Journal of Advanced Nursing* 8 (November 1983): 513–517.

Zappolo, A. "Discharge from Nursing Homes: 1977 National Nursing Home Survey." *Vital Health Statistics* 13 (August 1981): 1–75.

periodicals and other sources of information

The Coordinator
Coordinator Publications, Inc.
11417 Vanowen Street, North
Hollywood, CA 91605

Discharge Planning Update (quarterly newsletter)
AHA Services, Inc.
P.O. Box 99376
Chicago, IL 60693

Homecare Product Directory and Buyer's Guide
 (directory of products and meetings)
Miramar Publishing Company
2048 Cotner Avenue
Los Angeles, CA 90025

Homecare Product News (news and products information magazine)
Miramar Publishing Company
2048 Cotner Avenue
Los Angeles, CA 90025

Hospital Home Health (monthly newsletter)
67 Peachtree Park Drive, NE
Atlanta, GA 30309

Instructional Resources for Nurses
University of Michigan Media Library
R 4440 Kresge Box 56
Ann Arbor, MI 48109

Outreach (bimonthly report on ambulatory care,
 emergency services, health maintenance, home care,
 and hospice)
American Hospital Association
Division of Ambulatory Care
840 North Lake Shore Drive
Chicago, IL 60611

Publications and Audiovisual Aids List
National HomeCaring Council
235 Park Avenue South
New York, NY 10003

list of associations

Alzheimer's Disease and Related
  Disorders Association, Inc.
360 N. Michigan Avenue
Chicago, IL 60148
312/853-3060

American Association for
  Continuity of Care
1101 Connecticut Avenue
Suite 700
Washington, D.C. 20036
202/857-1194

American Association of Homes
  for the Aging
1050 17th Street N.W.
Suite 770
Washington, D.C. 20036
202/296-5960

American Association for
  Respiratory Therapy
1720 Regal Row
Dallas, TX 75235
214/630-3540

American Cancer Society, Inc.
777 Third Avenue
New York, NY 10017
212/371-2900

American Diabetes Association
Two Park Avenue
New York, NY 10016
212/683-7444

American Federation of Home Health
  Agencies, Inc.
429 N Street, S.W.
Suite 605
Washington, D.C. 20024
202/554-0526

American Health Care Association
1200 15th Street, N.W.
Washington, D.C. 20005
202/833-2050

American Heart Association
National Center
7320 Greenville Avenue
Dallas, TX 75231
214/750-5300

American Hospital Association
840 N. Lake Shore Drive
Chicago, IL 60611
312/280-6708

American Lung Association
1740 Broadway
New York, NY 10019
212/245-8000

American Medical Association
535 N. Dearborn Street
Chicago, IL 60610
312/645-5000

American Nurses' Association
2420 Pershing Road
Kansas City, MO 64108
816/474-5720

The American Occupational Therapy
  Association, Inc.
1383 Piccard Drive
Rockville, MD 20850
301/948-9626

American Pharmaceutical Association
2215 Constitution Avenue, N.W.
Washington, D.C. 20037
202/628-4411

American Physical Therapy Association
1111 North Fairfax Street
Alexandria, VA 22314
703/684-2782

American Society for Parenteral and
    Enteral Nutrition
1025 Vermont Avenue, N.E.
Suite 810
Washington, D.C. 20005
202/638-5881

American Red Cross
17th and D Streets, N.W.
Washington, D.C. 20006
202/737-8300

American Speech-Language-Hearing Association
10801 Rockville Pike
Rockville, MD 20852
301/897-5700

The Arthritis Foundation
1314 Spring Street, N.W.
Atlanta, GA 30309
404/872-7100

Association of Rehabilitation Nurses
2506 Grosse Point Road
Evanston, IL 60201
312/475-7530

Health Industry Manufacturers Association
1030 Fifteenth Street, N.W.
Suite 1100
Washington, D.C. 20005
202/452-8240

Home Health Services and Staffing Association
815 Connecticut Avenue, N.W.
Suite 206
Washington, D.C. 20006
202/331-4437

National Association of Boards of Examiners
    for Nursing Home Administrators, Inc.

45 N. Pennsylvania Street
Suite 612
Indianapolis, IN 46204
317/639-4387

National Association of Quality
    Assurance Professionals
1800 Pickwick Avenue
Glenview, IL 60025
312/724-7700

National Association of Social Workers
7981 Eastern Avenue
Silver Spring, MD 20910
202/565-0333

National Association for Home Care
519 C Street, N.E.
Washington, D.C. 20002
202/547-7424

National Council on the Aging, Inc.
600 Maryland Avenue, S.W.
Washington, D.C. 20024
202/479-1200

National Homecaring Council
235 Park Avenue South
New York, NY 10003
212/674-4990

National Hospice Organization
1901 N. Fort Myers Drive
Suite 402
Arlington, VA 22209
703/243-5900

National Kidney Foundation, Inc.
Two Park Avenue
New York, NY 10016
212/889-2210

National League for Nursing
10 Columbus Circle
New York, NY 10019
212/582-1022

Appendix A
STATISTICS FOR HISTORICAL REFERENCE

	1950	**1980s**
U.S. health care costs:	$12.7 billion, 4% GNP	$322 billion, 10.5% GNP
Medicare:	$56.8 billion (1970)	$565.6 billion (1984)
Medicaid:	since 1975, rising 18 percent a year.	

Liver transplant: $250,000

Kidney transplant: $18,000–$20,000

Coronary bypass: $16,000–$25,000

Source: Jack Star, "Putting a Clamp on Your Medical Costs," *Chicago*, June 1984, p. 166.

The health care component of the gross national product will increase from the present 10.5 percent to 12 percent by 1990.

Source: Hospital Week, August 17, 1984.

Costs of levels of care: $320 per month for rest home facility

$900 per month skilled nursing or extended care facility

$ 30 per visit for home care

$350 per day for acute-care hospital

$ 70 per day for nursing home care

$ 10 per day for foster home

Source: Susan Saul, *The Coordinator*, January 1984.

Total hospital admissions declined 2 percent to 8.94 million between the second and third quarters of 1984 (seasonally adjusted), the sharpest decline since admissions began to fall in the second quarter of 1983. This brings total admissions to the lowest quarterly level since 1978.

Source: Hospital Week, January 11, 1985

Admissions (second quarter of 1984): 1.6 percent decline

Length of stay: Patients under 65: 5.7 to 5.6 days

Patients over 65: 9.2 to 9.0 days

Source: Hospital Week, September 28, 1984.

Third-party coverage of home health care was virtually unheard of in 1970. Today, 65 percent of employers responding to a study conducted by Hewitt Associates (Illinois), are offering an increasing number of other nonhospital alternatives. Of 1,185 companies,

27% cover midwifery and birthing center services

36% cover hospice care

13% offer financial incentives to employees choosing hospice care

17% reimburse more fully for home care than for an extended inpatient stay

Source: Hospital Week, September 14, 1984.

Estimated number of home health agencies: 5,000. Of these, 3,800 are Medicare certified, 740 are for profit. In 1979 only 150 were for profit.

15 percent of not-for-profit hospitals offer home care services.

Source: Modern Healthcare, December 1983.

From the early part of the last century to the present, the factors predominantly responsible for improving life expectancy are:

1. Improved nutrition (70%).
2. Improved water systems and sanitation (20%).
3. All other factors, including reduced family size, immunization, and improved health care (10%).

Since 1900, only 6 percent of the improvement in life expectancy is attributed to medicine (such measures as antibiotics and life-saving surgery).

All current major causes of death are significantly affected by an individual's lifestyle:

Smoking and poor nutrition contribute to about 60–90 percent of cardiovascular disease; nutrition and smoking may play a role in 60–80 percent of cancer deaths; smoking contributes to about 50 percent of all respiratory disease; and consumption of alcohol plays a part in 50 percent of all accidental deaths.

Source: Robert E. McDermit, "The 'Wellness' Alternative," *Health Care*, June 1984.

Percentage of the U.S. population over 65 years old:

1900—4.0

1929—5.4

1940—6.8

1950—8.1

1960—9.2

2000—11.1 (estimate)

Source: U.S. Census Bureau.

---

7 percent of the aged are now institutionalized.

93 percent are not (and given an alternative, the majority may never need institutionalization).

Source: Hospitals, November 1, 1983.

Of America's 25.5 million senior citizens, 85 percent suffer from at least one chronic degenerative disease which, although it is not necessarily crippling, nevertheless diminishes personal independence and vitality.

Although elderly people make up less than 12 percent of population, they account for more than:

   25% of all prescriptions written

   33% of all occupied hospital beds

   30% of all health bills paid

Source: Ken Dychtwald, Ph.D., *Promoting Health*, September-October, 1984.

In 1979, about 40 percent of the nation's elderly were disabled to some degree.

Source: U.S. Department of Health, Education and Welfare.

25–40 percent of nursing home residents could be maintained at home if services such as food preparation, laundry, etc., could be provided. They are institutionalized because of lack of support services.

The most common home care diagnoses are:

   Circulatory disease

   Diabetes

   Cancer

   Other disabilities (inability to perform ADL, dysfunctional mental condition)

For example: 20% of patients are sometimes not alert

             60% need help walking

             90% need household assistance

Source: Mary Mundinger, *Home Health Care, too Little, Too Late, Too Costly.*

HCFA estimates that, on average, a person 65 or over spent a total of $4,202 in 1984 for health care services, including:

   $1,900 for hospital care

   $ 868 for physician services

   $ 880 for nursing home care

   $ 554 for prescription drugs

Source: Hospital Week, July 27, 1984.

The Greater New York Hospital Association states that there are 1,700 patients in the city awaiting nursing home placement. Costs: $350 per day in hospital as opposed to $75 per day in nursing home. Cost of inappropriate placement is $467,000 per day in New York City alone.

Source: Hospitals, March 16, 1984, p. 48.

The number of "homeless" people is estimated to be between 750,000 and 2,000,000.

Source: Betty Friedman, *Hospitals*, August 16, 1983.

One 1983 research study estimated that there were 3,000–4,000 homeless individuals in Atlanta. The homeless are defined as persons whose primary nighttime residences are streets, doorways of buildings, train and bus stations, parks, abandoned buildings, loading docks, public and private shelters for the homeless, and similar sites.

Source: The American Nurse, February 1, 1985.

A 20-state study of ventilator patients carried out by the American Association of Respiratory Therapy shows that many are institutionalized for financial reasons. The study reviewed 2,272 ventilator-dependent patients in hospitals. Of these, 258 are deemed medically able to go home (16 percent were under age 17).

Inpatient costs: $270,000 per patient per year

Home care costs: $21,192 per patient per year

Possible savings: $64.4 million

Source: Home Health Care Journal, April 1, 1984.

Appendix B
GLOSSARY

Acute disease. A disease of short duration, usually less than one month (single episode), from which the individual is expected to recover to his or her pre-disease state.

Alternative care. Any setting for care other than the acute-care hospital; also refers to types of medical care, such as nutrition therapy.

Care plan. A formal written plan of activities to be conducted by personnel of a long term care facility, home health agency, hospital, or other health facility on behalf of a patient and to be used to evaluate that patient's needs and progress.

Client. See **Patient**.

Coinsurance. The insurance company pays a portion of the cost of the services or care and the subscriber pays the balance.

Consumer. See **Patient**.

Coordination of benefits. A provision for nonduplication of benefits when two or more organizations provide similar health care coverage.

Coverage. The extent of benefits provided under a contract.

Deductible. The amount of expense a subscriber must incur before receiving contract benefits; the subscriber must pay the deductible amount.

Diagnosis related group (DRG). A classification system that groups patients into categories based on the following variables: diagnosis, age, treatment, surgery, complications, comorbid conditions, length of stay.

Discharge coordinator. The person who arranges with health or community agencies and institutions to engage in the care of patients upon discharge from a hospital.

Discharge planning. Centralized, coordinated program developed by a hospital to ensure that each patient has a planned program for needed continuing or follow-up care.

Discharge referral. A written or verbal communication sent from one care setting to another that informs personnel of a patient's need for continued care.

Discharge transfer. The disposition of a patient to another health care institution at time of discharge from the inpatient setting for continued care or rehabilitation.

Durable medical equipment (DME). Items of medical equipment that have been ordered by the physician for the care of the patient. Their costs may or may not be reimbursable under Medicare and Medicaid. Medicare has a handbook for covered items, and Medicaid may cover some with prior approval.

ECF. Extended care facility.

Family. Used here to include the patient's main support persons. It may or may not include the patient's biological family. It may include or be limited to those individuals frequently referred to as "significant others," such as a friend, neighbor, roommate, or co-worker.

HCFA. Health Care Financing Administration.

Health maintenance organization (HMO). An organization that provides, on a prepayment basis, a comprehensive range of health care services for the subscriber, who is voluntarily enrolled. Emphasis is on preventive care rather than crisis-oriented care; the HMO "profits" by keeping the subscriber well and out of the hospital or other institution.

HHS. Department of Health and Human Services. Formerly HEW, the Department of Health, Education and Welfare.

Financially institutionalized. Refers to patients hospitalized because reimbursement is available for hospital care but not for home care for the patient's particular condition.

Home health aide. An individual who has been trained to work under the supervision of a registered nurse to carry out activities related to daily living needs, such as: bathing, personal hygiene, turning/lifting/transfer, ambulation, prescribed simple exercises (ROM), and limited household tasks. The aide may not dispense medications but may remind a patient to take them.

Home care. The component of comprehensive health care whereby services are provided to individuals and families in their places of residence for the purposes of promoting, maintaining, or restoring health or minimizing the effects of illness and disability. Services appropriate to the needs of the individual patient and family are planned, coordinated, and made available by an agency or institution, organized for the delivery of health care through the use of employed staff, contractual arrangements, or a combination of administrative personnel. These services are provided under a plan of care that includes services such as, but not limited to, medical care, dental care, nursing, physical therapy, speech therapy, occupational therapy, social work, nutrition, homemaker or home health aide, transportation, laboratory services, medical equipment, and supplies.

Home health agency (HHA). An agency whose specialty is providing care to patients at home. Depending on the location and intent of the agency, it may or may not be Medicare approved or licensed by the state (not all states require licensure). There are seven services usually offered by home health agencies: nursing (skilled, intermittent), home health aides, physical therapy, occupational therapy, speech therapy, medical social work, and hospice. Other services, such as nutrition counseling, respiratory care, laboratory and X-ray, podiatry, spiritual care, supplies and equipment, and dental care, may also be provided. Homemaking, meals, transportation, housekeeping, and other such services are usually referred to as supportive services and may or may not be part of an agency's services; generally, they are not.

ICD-9-CM. *International Classification of Diseases, 9th ed., Clinical Modification.*

MCD. Major diagnostic category.

ICF. Intermediate care facility.

Liaison nurse. Often a member of the hospital or nursing home discharge planning staff who serves as a link between the institution and other community health care centers to ensure continuity of care.

LOS. Length of stay: number of days a patient is in an institution as an inpatient.

Medicaid. Title XIX (Public Law 87-97), Medical Assistance, Amendment to the Social Security Act of 1965. Provides a program of care for public aid recipients and people whose income exceeds public aid limits but who meet other criteria and cannot pay for medical services.

Medicare. Title XVIII (Public Law 87-97), Health Insurance for the Aged, Amendment to the Social Security Act of 1965. Provides a program of medical care for persons age 65 and over and selected persons under 65. Includes two programs of health insurance protection: Hospital insurance (Part A), which covers hospitalization and related care; and medical insurance (Part B), which covers physician's care and other health services. Both Parts A and B have some specific provisions for home care.

NAEHCA. National Association of Employees on Health Care Alternatives.

Nursing care plan. Data concerning a specific patient that is organized in a concise and systematic manner, that facilitates the achievement of medical and nursing goals, and that clearly states the nature of the patient's problems and the related medical and nursing orders. Identifies patient problems, expected outcomes, and prescribed nursing actions.

PAT. Preadmission testing: performance of needed tests in the hospital before actual hospital admission. Purpose is to decrease the length of stay and to prevent unnecessary hospitalization. For example, testing of a preoperative patient may indicate the presence of infection and thus prevent the admission of the patient until the condition is treated and cleared.

Patient. Term used interchangeably with **client** and **consumer** to indicate the individual who is in need of the assistance of a health care giver for resolution of an identified health care problem.

PPS. Prospective payment system: A system wherein the method of payment by third-party payers is based on predetermined estimates made at the beginning of a fiscal period and not based on actual costs (the opposite of the traditional cost-based, fee-for-service method of reimbursement). As of October 1, 1983, prospective payment for recipients of Medicare is in effect and reimbursement is determined by diagnosis related groups (DRGs).

Premature discharge. A "too early" discharge with regard to the patient's medical condition and care needs. Not synonymous with *early discharge.*

PRO. Professional review organization.

PSRO. Professional standards review organization: A Medicare, Medicaid, and maternal and child health program administered on a regional basis, centering on physician-sponsored care review and audit and often tied into reimbursement for patient services.

Reasonable and customary charges. An indefinable term.

Section 223. A part of the Social Security Amendments of 1972 that HHS to establish limits on overall direct or indirect costs that will be recognized as reasonable under Medicare for comparable services in comparable facilities in an area.

Skilled nursing. Services that must be rendered by a registered nurse to achieve the medically desired results and to ensure the safety of the patient.

TEFRA. Tax Equity and Fiscal Responsibility Act of 1982 (Public Law 97-248). Laid the groundwork for PPS, which was put into operation for Medicare recipients on October 1, 1983.

Timely fashion. An indefinable term.

UB-82. The Uniform Bill (National Uniform Billing) intended to be used by the major third-party payers, most hospitals (for inpatient and outpatient billing), and, at the option of the hospital, hospital-based skilled nursing facilities and home health agencies.

UR. Utilization review: the process of examining the efficiency of institutional use, the appropriateness of admissions, services ordered and provided, length of stay, and discharge practices on both a concurrent and retrospective basis.

Appendix C
DISCHARGE PLANNING GUIDELINES, JOB DESCRIPTIONS, AND FORMS

COMPONENTS OF A DISCHARGE PLANNING PROGRAM

by Garnett Jones

Structure

Philosophy
Goals
Organizational framework
Responsibility, accountability
Objectives
Policies and procedures
Discharge planning committee

Process

Problem identification
Referral
Physician involvement
Patient/family involvement
Interdisciplinary coordination
Problem clarification
Case conferences
Final discharge plan
Implementation
Evaluation

Outcomes

Patient satisfaction
Community perception
Length of stay
Cost effectiveness
Effectiveness of the process

GUIDELINES: DISCHARGE PLANNING

Introduction

The American Hospital Association believes that coordinated discharge planning functions are essential for hospitals to maintain high-quality patient care. Discharge planning is important because it facilitates appropriate patient and family decision making. In addition, it can also help reduce length of stay and the rate of increase of health care costs.

For most patients, discharge planning is a part of routine patient care. For those patients whose posthospital needs are expected to be complex, special discharge planning services are warranted. These guidelines present general information for organizing services for complex discharge planning.

It is recognized that each hospital has different resources and organizes its services differently to meet specific patient needs. It is further recognized that rapid changes in the hospital environment cause rapid changes in discharge planning. These changes, however, have emphasized the importance of discharge planning, and it is in that context that these guidelines are presented.

Definition

Discharge planning is an interdisciplinary hospital-wide process that should be available to aid patients and their families in developing a feasible posthospital plan of care.

Purposes

The purposes of discharge planning are to ensure the continuity of high-quality patient care, the availability of the hospital's resources for other patients requiring admission, and the appropriate utilization of resources. To ensure the continuity of high-quality care, the hospital will:

- Assign responsibility for the coordination of discharge planning
- Identify as early as possible, sometimes before hospital admission, the expected posthospital care needs of patients utilizing admission and preadmission and screening and review programs when available
- Develop with patients and their families appropriate discharge care plans

- Assist patients and their families in planning for the supportive environment necessary to provide the patients' posthospital care
- Develop a plan that considers the medical, social, and financial needs of patients

To ensure the availability of hospital resources for subsequent patients with due regard for prospective pricing, the hospital's procedures should be carried out in such a manner as to accomplish timely discharge.

Principles of Discharge Planning

The discharge planning process incorporates a determination of the patient's posthospital care preferences, needs, the patient's capacity for self-care, an assessment of the patient's living conditions, the identification of health or social care resources needed to assure high-quality posthospital care, and the counseling of the patient or family to prepare them for posthospital care. Discharge planning should be carried out in keeping with varying community resources and hospital utilization activities.

Discharge Planning when Multiple Resources are Required

In addition to discharge instructions for each routine patient discharge plan, the coordination of multiple resources may be required to achieve continued safe and high-quality posthospital care in situations where the patient's needs are complicated.

Essential Elements

The essential elements in accomplishing the hospital's goals for high-quality, cost-effective patient care are:

• Early Identification of Patients Likely to Need Complex Posthospital Care

There are certain factors that may indicate a need for early initiation of discharge planning, either before admission or upon admission. Screens for automatic early patient identification are developed for each specialty service by the physician and relevant health care providers and used as guidelines to carry out discharge planning.

• Patient and Family Education

With greater emphasis on self-care, patient and

family education is critical to successful discharge planning. The coordination of discharge planning must integrate teaching about physical care to facilitate approprite self-care in the home.

• Patient/Family Assessment and Counseling

The psychosocial and physical assessment and counseling of patients and families to determine the full range of needs upon discharge and to prepare them for the posthospital stage of care is a dynamic process. This process includes evaluation of the patient's and the family's strengths and weaknesses; the patient's physical condition; understanding the illness and treatment; the ability to assess the patient's and family capacities to adapt to changes; and, where necessary, to assist the persons involved to manage in their continued care. Discharge planning and the coordination of posthospital care plans requires an ability to adapt the plans to meet changes in the patient's condition.

• Plan Development

The discharge plan development should include the results of the assessment and the self-care instructions, including information from the patient, the family, and all relevant health care professionals. Service needs and options are identified, and the patient and family are helped to under-

stand the consequences of whatever plan they choose to adopt. A supportive climate is critical to facilitate appropriate decision making.

• Plan Coordination and Implementation

The hospital achieves high-quality and effective discharge planning through the delegation of specific responsibilities to the principal and specialized disciplines providing care. In order to minimize the potential for fragmented care and to fulfill the need for a central hospital linkage to the community, there should be assigned responsibility for discharge planning coordination for complex cases.

• Postdischarge Follow-Up

In complex situations requiring coordinated discharge planning, the plans should ensure follow-up with the patient, the family, and/or community service(s) providing continued care to determine the discharge plan outcome.

Quality Assurance

The quality of the discharge planning system should be monitored through the hospitalwide quality assurance program.

© 1984 by the American Hospital Association, 840 North Lake Shore Drive, Chicago, Illinois, 60611. All rights reserved. Reprinted by permission of the American Hospital Association.

ADMISSION ASSESSMENT AND NURSING NOTES

<table>
<tr><td rowspan="4">ADMISSIONS</td><td>DATE</td><td>TIME</td><td>☐ A.M.
☐ P.M.</td><td colspan="2">IDENTIFICATION BRACELET CHECKED?</td><td>☐ YES   ☐ NO</td></tr>
<tr><td colspan="6">MODE OF ADMISSION: ☐ WALKING   ☐ WHEELCHAIR   ☐ STRETCHER   ☐ OTHER:</td></tr>
<tr><td colspan="6">ACCOMPANIED BY: ☐ UNACCOMPANIED</td></tr>
<tr><td colspan="6">☐ PRIMARY LANGUAGE: ☐ ENGLISH   ☐ SPANISH   ☐ OTHER: INFORMATION FROM WHOM?</td></tr>
</table>

CONSENT | **X, IF SIGNED** > ☐ FOR MEDICAL TREATMENT   ☐ RELEASE OF RESPONSIBILITY OF VALUABLES

SOCIAL ASSESSMENT | OCCUPATION   RELIGIOUS PREFERENCE   HEALTH EDUCATION CLASSES ATTENDED

HOME CARE ASSESSMENT

WITH WHOM DO YOU LIVE? | DO YOU HAVE ANY DEPENDENTS? | ARE ANY OF THEM DISABLED? | IF "YES" DESCRIBE

IF "YES" HOW MANY?   ☐ YES   ☐ NO   ☐ YES   ☐ NO

WHERE DO YOU LIVE? > ☐ HOUSE ☐ APARTMENT   ☐ FOSTER CARE HOME   DO YOU HAVE TO CLIMB STAIRS? ☐ YES ☐ NO
☐ ROOM ☐ HEALTH CARE FACILITY   ☐ OTHER (DESCRIBE):

IS THERE A BATHROOM ON THE MAIN FLOOR? ☐ YES ☐ NO | IS IT NEAR WHERE YOU SLEEP? ☐ YES ☐ NO | HAVE YOU EVER UTILIZED ANY OF THE FOLLOWING TO RECUPERATE IN THE PAST? ☐ NO ☐ NURSING HOME ☐ VISITING NURSE IN YOUR HOME ☐ OTHER:

DO YOU HAVE SOME ONE TO ASSIST YOU AFTER DISCHARGE, IF NECESSARY? ☐ YES ☐ NO > IF "YES", NAME:

ADDRESS, CITY, STATE, ZIP   PHONE NUMBER

DO YOU HAVE SPECIAL EQUIPMENT AT HOME? ☐ NONE | ANY ADDITIONAL EQUIPMENT NEEDED?
☐ WHEELCHAIR ☐ WALKER ☐ COMMODE ☐ OTHER: | ☐ YES ☐ NO   IF "YES" LIST:

VALUABLES AND/OR MONEY | ☐ NONE   ☐ SENT HOME   ☐ TO CASHIER > DESCRIBE:

EXPLANATIONS

☐ PER VOLUNTEER: | ☐ ADMISSIONS KIT | ☐ CALL SYSTEM | ☐ VISITING POLICIES | ☐ BED OPERATION | ☐ TELEVISION
| ☐ BATHROOM FACILITIES | ☐ SELECTIVE MENUS | ☐ MAIL DELIVERIES | ☐ MEAL HOURS | ☐ TELEPHONE

HISTORY OF PRESENT ILLNESS

REASON FOR HOSPITALIZATION: FAMILY DOCTOR

SYMPTOMS AND TREATMENT BEFORE HOSPITALIZATION:

DID THE DOCTOR TELL YOU HE/SHE IS GOING TO ORDER ANY SPECIAL TESTS?   ☐ YES ☐ NO | TESTS

PAST SURGERIES AND HOSPITALIZATIONS

CHRONIC ILLNESSES

SYSTEMS REVIEW

E.E.N.T.

☐ EYE GLASSES	☐ BLINDNESS	☐ INFLAMATION	☐ NO SIGNIFICANT FINDINGS	DESCRIBE:
☐ CONTACT LENS	☐ BLURRING	☐ PROSTHESIS		
☐ DEAF	☐ HOH (L)	☐ TINNITUS	DESCRIBE:	
☐ HEARING AIDE	☐ HOH (R)	☐ NO SIGN. FINDINGS		
☐ HOARSENESS	☐ PAIN	☐ NO SIGNIFICANT FINDINGS	DESCRIBE:	
☐ STOMATITIS	☐ DRAINAGE			

FORM NO. NS 520.30 (REV. 6/83)

ADMISSION ASSESSMENT and NURSING NOTES

<table>
<tr><td rowspan="2">RESPIRATORY ASSESSMENT</td><td colspan="5">☐ DYSPNEA   ☐ CYANOSIS   ☐ CONGESTION   ☐ SMOKES</td></tr>
</table>

RESPIRATORY ASSESSMENT

☐ DYSPNEA ☐ CYANOSIS ☐ CONGESTION ☐ SMOKES

☐ O²   LITERS: MODE   COUGH ⟩ ☐ PRODUCTIVE ☐ NONPRODUCTIVE ☐ NO SIGNIFICANT FINDINGS

DESCRIBE:

LUNG SOUNDS:

CARDIO-VASCULAR

☐ EDEMA   ☐ CHEST PAIN   ☐ HYPERTENSION   ☐ OTHER:

IRREGULAR PULSE: ☐ A/R _____   ☐ NVD   **EXTREMITIES** ⟩ ☐ COOL ☐ WARM ☐ DISCOLORED ☐ NO SIGNIFICANT FINDING

DESCRIBE:

IF ALTERATIONS IN EXTREMITY ASSESSMENT PRESENT, FURTHER ASSESSMENT SHOULD INCLUDE:

		RIGHT	LEFT			RIGHT	LEFT
EXTREMITY PULSES ⟩	RADIAL:			BRACHIAL:			

DORSALIS PEDIS:	RIGHT	LEFT	POSTERIOR TIBIAL:	RIGHT	LEFT	OTHER (SPECIFY)	RIGHT	LEFT

NEURO-MUSCULAR SKELETAL

☐ HEADACHES ☐ ROM LIMITATIONS   ORIENTATION: PERSON   PLACE   TIME   ☐ PERL ☐ PROSTHESIS

☐ SPEECH IMPAIRMENT ☐ GAIT IMPAIRMENTS   ☐ MISSING LIMBS

☐ NO SIGNIFICANT FINDINGS   DESCRIBE   ☐ MORE THOROUGH ASSESSMENT NEEDED—USE NEUROLOGY NURSING ASSESSMENT

G.I. (BOWEL ASSESSMENT)

☐ CONSTIPATION ☐ DISTENDED ABDOMEN ☐ HEMORRHOIDS   ABNORMAL STOOLS: COLOR   CONSISTENCY   SHAPE   CHARACTER

☐ DIARRHEA ☐ OSTOMY ☐ INCONTINENT

BOWEL SOUNDS-DESCRIBE: NORMAL BOWEL FUNCTION

AIDS TO ELIMINATION   LAST B.M.   DESCRIBE FINDINGS

G.I. (NUTRITION)

☐ UPPER DENTURES   SPECIAL DIET

☐ LOWER DENTURES

☐ PARTIAL PLATE   SPECIAL EATING HABITS

☐ DYSPHAGIA

☐ NAUSEA   SUPPLEMENTAL NOURISHMENT   ALCOHOL USE

☐ NO SIGNIFICANT FINDINGS

☐ OTHER: DESCRIBE FINDINGS:

WHEN ANY OF THE FOLLOWING EXISTS, A DIETARY CONSULT IS NECESSARY

☐ RECENT 10% WEIGHT LOSS OR GAIN

☐ PREGNANCY

☐ OVER 60/TEENAGER

☐ CHEMO/RADIATION TREATMENT

☐ DENTAL PROBLEMS

☐ MULTIPLE DISEASE STATES (ACUTE AND CHRONIC)

G.U.

☐ BURNING ☐ NOCTURIA ☐ CATHETER   ☐ NO. SIGN. FINDINGS   LMP   PARA   GRAVIDA   PAP SMEAR

☐ ITCHING ☐ ABNORMAL URINE ☐ INCONTINENT

☐ URGENCY ☐ BIRTH CONTROL ☐ ODOR   DESCRIBE:

☐ FREQUENCY ☐ MENSES ☐ DISCHARGE

PHYSICAL FINDINGS

FAMILIAR WITH SELF BREAST EXAM ☐ YES ☐ NO

PRACTICES MONTHLY ☐ YES ☐ NO

☐ (1) BRUISES ☐ (4) ULCERATIONS ☐ (7) NUMBNESS ☐ (10) PARALYSIS

☐ (2) RASHES ☐ (5) INCISIONS ☐ (8) TINGLING ☐ (11) ABNORMAL COLOR

☐ (3) SCARS ☐ (6) DECUBITUS ☐ (9) WEAKNESS ☐ (12) ABNORMAL TURGOR

DESCRIBE (GRAPH ALL IDENTIFIED ALTERATIONS):   ☐ NO. SIGN. FINDINGS

FRONT   **BACK**

EMOTIONAL STATUS

ADDITIONAL ADMISSION NOTES ON 24 HOUR NURSING RECORD ☐ YES ☐ NO

ADMISSION PROBLEM LIST (TRANSFER TO CARE PLAN)

NURSING SIGNATURES

L.P.N.   DATE   R.N.   DATE

TIME ☐ A.M. ☐ P.M.   TIME ☐ A.M. ☐ P.M.

By permission of Edward W. Sparrow Hospital Association, Lansing, Michigan.

REFERRAL FOR CONTINUITY OF PATIENT CARE
(HOSPITAL-EXTENDED CARE FACILITY-HOME HEALTH SERVICE)

Transfer From	Transfer To	Social Security No.

Sex	Age	Birth Date	Phone	Marital Status	Religion	Date Adm.	Date Trans.

Medicare Claim No.	Other insurance coverage	Social Agency Active

Physician in charge	Physician in charge after trans.	Case Worker

Is patient or family aware of diagnosis?
Patient: ☐ Yes ☐ No Family: ☐ Yes ☐ No

Estimated Medicare days left this spell of illness:
Hospital _____ Ext. Care Fac. _____

Name and address of responsible relative or guardian:
Phone_____

Address patient was transferred (if different from above)

Diagnosis Primary (operation or delivery date) | Other diagnosis (including pertinent past history & sensitivities)

Transfer orders of physician
(Including medications, dosages & treatments)

DIET:
Regular _____
Diabetic _____
Low Salt _____
Low Res. _____
Soft _____
Other _____

OTHER SERVICES REQUIRED:
(Specify under transfer order)
Physical Therapy _____
Occupational Therapy _____
Speech Therapy _____
Home Health Aide _____
Medical Social Worker _____
Dietician _____

TESTS GIVEN: DATE: RESULTS:
___ Chest X-Ray _____ _____
___ PPD _____ _____
___ Serology _____ _____
___ Blood Sugar _____ _____
___ Other _____ _____

DISABILITIES:
Amputations___ Paralysis___
Contractures___ Decubitus___
IMPAIRMENTS:
Speech___ Vision___
Hearing___ Sensation___
INCONTINENCE:
Bladder___ Bowel___

PATIENT CAN TRAVEL TO CLINIC OR OFFICE BY:
Ambulance_____
Car _____
Bus _____
Other _____

SUGGESTIONS FOR ACTIVE CARE:
BED: Prone position___times per day as tolerated.
Avoid___ position___ change position every____ hours.
SIT: In chair___ Hrs.___ Time per day: stand___ mins.___ times___
Per day: walk___ times per day.
WEIGHT BEARING: Full___ Partial___ None___ On___ Leg
EXERCISES: Range of motion___ times per day

ORAL HEALTH (include dental conditions & treatment necessary):

SELF CARE STATUS: if relevant, indicate if
a) needs supervision; b) needs assistance; c) needs instruction, d) unable to do; or e) independent.
LANGUAGE: understands English _____
speaks English _____
MENTAL STATUS: Alert _____ Withdrawn _____
Aggressive _____ Confused _____
PERSONAL CARE:
Bathing _____ Dressing _____
Feeding _____
LOCOMOTION: Walking _____ Wheelchair _____
BED: Turning _____ Sitting _____
ELIMINATION: Bladder ___ Bowel ___ Saliva _____
Comments: _____

CERTIFICATION: I certify that the transfer of the above patient to
(Hospital), (Extended Care Facility), (Home Health Service) is
necessary for the continuing treatment of the diagnosis listed:

_____   _____
(Date)   (Physician)

REPORT OF STAFF NURSE, PHYSICAL THERAPIST, SOCIAL WORKER, DIETITIAN, ETC. (Include summary of patient's progress,
significant nursing care plans or assessments by other personnel; socio-economic problems; patient's discharge
status and supplies available).

Agency & Person Contacted   Title   Referring Agent   Title   Date

REFERRAL FOR CONTINUITY OF PATIENT CARE

SUPPLEMENTAL SHEET

CHECK PURPOSE FOR WHICH FORM IS BEING USED:

☐ INFORMATION REQUEST

☐ ADDITIONAL INFORMATION
   Continuation of referral form and report of other
   staff -- Social Service, Dietary, OT, PT -- include
   observations, results of teaching, environmental,
   cultural or financial problems, plans made, etc.

☐ REPORT FROM HOME HEALTH SERVICE, OR SNF
   Include patient's condition, care and instruction
   given, home and family situation. Describe plans
   for further care; include district, telephone
   number, and date of visit.

FROM_____
        (Name of facility or agency)

TO_____
        (Name of facility or agency)
(Add signature, title & date after each entry)

ROUTING COPIES: White = Nursing Home with Ambulance Driver, Home Health to Social Service Department;
          Yellow = on chart; Pink = To Social Services; Gold = To Social Services.

By permission of Silver Cross Hospital, Joliet, Illinois.

DISCHARGE PLANNING IN THE NEONATAL INTENSIVE CARE SETTING

by Christa Harp, RN

The discharge process should begin when the patient enters the health care system. Admission to an ICU is usually sudden and anxiety provoking. Early supportive contact by reassuring staff members is required. Distortion of information commonly occurs; therefore, frequent explanations and interpretations are needed to provide the family with reality-based information. This need for knowledge continues throughout the patient's hospitalization and becomes even more acute as discharge approaches.

The family of the neonatal ICU patient is especially vulnerable to emotional trauma and requires ongoing assessment, support, and opportunity to meet with staff members. The parents become the extended care facility and the focus of patient education. Their learning needs have to be met throughout the baby's hospitalization. Early participation in preparation for discharge allows the parents to phase themselves in as the caretakers and to assume as much responsibility for the infant as possible. Education encourages the growth of the parents' confidence in their caretaking skills and helps them view the infant's potential needs realistically.

The family participates in discharge planning by being involved in the design of realistic goals. Both long-term and short-term goals are set, and the parents are helped to find ways to fulfill them. Understanding the hows and whys of care is fundamental to maintaining and increasing the well-being of the infant in the home. Family involvement in goal setting also increases the potential for compliance.

An important element of discharge planning is the assessment and counseling carried out by the social worker to determine the family's needs, strengths, and weaknesses. The social worker, an integral part of the interdisciplinary team involved in discharge planning, assists the family by counseling them about financial matters, communication problems, mobility, and special discharge services needed. Evaluation of the effectiveness of the plan is done by follow-up several months after discharge to make sure that the discharge was not premature.

Discharge Checklist

General care discharge

A. *Nutrition*

Infant

____ *1.   Weight approximately 2 kilograms.
____ 2.   Steady weight gain of 10-15 gm per day.
____ 3.   Well established on p.o. feedings; tolerating feedings.

Parents

____ 1.   Able to feed (breast or bottle).
____ 2.   Able to prepare formula.
____ 3.   Able to assess appropriateness of intake and output.

*Check (✔) if completed; write "NA" if not applicable

B. *Health care maintenance*

Infant

____ 1. Able to maintain body temperature in an open crib.
____ 2. All laboratory test results within normal limits.
____ 3. Necessary screening completed:
  a. Newborn metabolic screening or plans for follow-up.
  b. Ophthalmology exam.
  c. Audiology exam.
____ 4. Weaned off as many medications as possible with time to evaluate the effects on the infant.

Parents

____ 1. Able to bathe and dress infant, perform cord and circumcision care.
____ 2. Know how to use bulb syringe.
____ 3. Able to take infant's rectal temperature and keep infant in a state of good temperature control.
____ 4. Knowledgeable about infant sleeping habits.
____ 5. Able to administer medications appropriately.
____ 6. Aware of common illnesses and their treatment.
____ 7. Know CPR skills.
____ 8. Acquainted with the use of a car seat.
____ 9. Able to administer medications appropriately.

C. *Follow-up*

____ 1. Clinic or private pediatrician.
____ 2. PHN as required.
____ 3. Discharge summary for follow-up physician.
____ 4. Audiology, ophthalmology follow-up if needed.

In addition to general discharge care, the chronically ill infant has specialized needs.

Chronic care discharge

A. *Nutrition*

____ 1. Gavage feeding instructions and performance, if necessary.
____ 2. Dietitian consult.

A. *Medications*

Infant

____ 1. Consistent dose and route of medication administration for one week.
____ 2. Adequate time after beginning or discontinuing a drug to monitor its effects on the infant.

Parents

____ 1. Feel comfortable with medication administration.
____ 2. Know signs and symptoms of toxicity.
____ 3. Have available needed equipment for administration.
____ 4. Written instructions for medication administration if medications are numerous.
____ 5. Know what action to take if infant vomits medications.

C. *Pulmonary care*

Infant

____ 1.   Consistent blood gas readings for at least one week.
____ 2.   Consistent FIO_2 levels and delivery system (nasal cannula) for one week.
____ 3.   Stable respiratory status (i.e., no significant apnea).
____ 4.   Cardiac monitor if occasionally apneic; or abnormal sleep study.
____ 5.   Sleep study.

Parents

____ 1.   Familiar and comfortable with O_2 delivery system.
____ 2.   Have a reliable source for obtaining and maintaining equipment in their community.
____ 3.   Have portable and back-up O_2 delivery systems.
____ 4.   Have appropriate amounts of additional supplies (cannulas, suction catheters, etc.).
____ 5.   Are able to identify times of increased O_2 needs and signs of deteriorating pulmonary status.
____ 6.   Know how to perform CPT, percussion, and postural drainage.
____ 7.   Have a resource person at the University to contact in case of an emergency (neonatologist or pulmonologist).

Follow-up

____ 1.   Pulmonologist.
____ 2.   Specialty clinics.

Source: University Hospital, University of Utah Health Sciences Center. Used by permission.

INFANT DISCHARGE RECORD

						PATIENT CASE NUMBER	
1 REFERRING HOSPITAL NAME	HOSP. CODE	PERINATAL CENTER NAME				CTR. CODE	PATIENT ID. NUMBER
2 INFANT'S LAST NAME	FIRST NAME		M.I.	DATE OF BIRTH		FAMILY CASE NO. (IDPH USE ONLY)	
3 DATE OF ADMISSION	RACE ☐ WHITE ☐ BLACK ☐ ORIENTAL			SEX ☐ M ☐ F		COUNTY OF RESIDENCE	CNTY. CODE
4 MOTHERS LAST NAME	FIRST NAME		M.I.	DATE OF BIRTH		TELEPHONE NUMBER ( )	
5 MOTHERS STREET ADDRESS — APT. NUMBER		CITY		STATE			ZIP CODE

6 MOTHERS MAIDEN NAME	MARITAL STATUS ☐ MARRIED ☐ UNMARRIED	PERINATAL SOCIAL WORKER NAME	TELEPHONE
7 FATHERS LAST NAME	FIRST NAME	REFERRING PHYSICIAN NAME	
8 ATTENDING PHYSICIAN AT PERINATAL CENTER		NURSE CONTACT AT PERINATAL CENTER	TELEPHONE

9 DISCHARGE DATE	DISCHARGED ALIVE ☐ YES ☐ NO	DATE OF DEATH	CAUSE OF DEATH

10 IF DISCHARGED ALIVE, COMPLETE THE REST OF THIS FORM

11 DISCHARGE WEIGHT _____ GRAMS	DISCHARGE HEAD CIRCUMFERENCE _____ CM	ASSISTED VENTILATION _____ O$_2$ONLY _____ CPAP _____ RESP	INFANT PLACED OUTSIDE OF FAMILY? ☐ YES ☐ NO
		COMMENTS	

12 PARENTS PARTICIPATION/INTERACTION
☐ EXCELLENT ☐ GOOD ☐ FAIR ☐ NONE

13 BREAST FEEDING ☐ YES ☐ NO   BOTTLE FEEDING   FREQUENCY_____ AMOUNT_____ FORMULA_____

14 SPECIFIC FEEDING PROBLEMS / INSTRUCTIONS

15 DISCHARGE DIAGNOSIS AND CONDITION

16

17 SPECIFIC DISCHARGE TREATMENTS

18

19 OTHER CONCERNS (HEALTH, SOCIAL, DEVELOPMENTAL, ETC.)

20

22 CONTACT PERSON NAME (OTHER THAN PARENT)	RELATIONSHIP	TELEPHONE NUMBER
23 STREET ADDRESS	CITY	ZIP CODE

24 FAMILY INFORMED OF LOCAL HEALTH NURSE VISIT? ☐ YES _____ DATE	CURRENT SOCIAL SERVICES		
25 LHN AGENCY NAME	STREET ADDRESS	CITY	ZIP CODE CODE

SIGNATURES_____

_____

DATE_____

By permission of Illinois Department of Public Health, Perinatal Center.

113

INFANT REPORT (REPORT OF PUBLIC HEALTH NURSE)

INFANT REPORT	REPORT OF PUBLIC HEALTH NURSE		PATIENT CASE NUMBER	
INFANTS LAST NAME	FIRST NAME	MI	DATE OF BIRTH	
STREET ADDRESS	CITY		DATE OF VISIT	VISIT NUMBER	PREDISCHARGE VISIT MADE ☐ YES ☐ NO
PUBLIC HEALTH AGENCY NAME		AGENCY CODE	PHYSICIAN NAME	CASE CLOSED ☐ YES

PHYSICAL APPRAISAL			DEVELOPMENTAL SCREENING					
HEAD CIRCUMFERENCE _____ CM			PLEASE PERFORM SCREEN APPROPRIATELY FOR CHRONOLOGICAL AND ADJUSTED AGE					
CHECK APPROPRIATE BOX			RSA FROM BIRTH	PRES-ENT	AB-SENT	RSA BY 9 MONTHS	PRES-ENT	AB-SENT
INAPPROPRIATE			REGARDS FACE			SITS ALONE WELL		
			MOVEMENTS OF ALL EXTREMITIES, BILATERAL AND SYMMETRICAL			PULLS UP ON FURNITURE		
APPROPRIATE						PICKS UP PENNY WITH THUMB/FORE FINGER GRASP		
GENERAL APPEARANCE			RESPONDS TO SOUND (USUALLY BLINKS, WIDENS EYELIDS, MOMENTARILY CEASES ACTIVITY OR STARTLES)			IMITATES SOUNDS OR WORDS		
HEAD						PLAYS PEEK-A-BOO OR BYE-BYE		
EYES			PLACING			TONIC NECK REFLEX DISAPPEARED		
NOSE			STEPPING			HEAD UP, BACK ARCHED ON VENTRAL SUSPENSION (LANDAU)		
MOUTH			RSA BY 6 WEEKS			TURNS HEAD TO SOUND		
CHEST			EYES FOLLOW 90° (E.G. FACE, SPARKLER, RED RING)			RSA BY 12 MONTHS		
CARDIOVASCULAR						WALKS, ONE HAND HELD		
ABDOMEN			MAKES THROATY NOISES			TRANSFERS OBJECTS		
GENITALIA			WHEN PRONE (ON STOM.) LIFTS HEAD BRIEF			ONE WORD OTHER THAN MAMA OR DADA		
			GRASPS EXAMINER'S FINGER			IMITATES RATTLING SPOON IN CUP		
BACK			SMILES RESPONSIVELY			PLAYS PAT-A-CAKE		
			RESPONDS TO SOUND			EXTENDS HANDS AND ARMS DEFENSIVELY WHEN THREATENED HEAD FIRST (PARACHUTE)		
EXTREMITIES			RSA BY 3 MONTHS					
HIPS			HELD SITTING, HOLDS HEAD ERECT BRIEFLY			TURNS HEAD TO SOUND		
SKIN			HANDS OPEN OR RELAXED; HOLDS EXAMINER'S FINGER AND WON'T LET GO			RSA BY 15 MONTHS		
NEUROLOGICAL						WALKS ALONE		
TONE / STRENGTH			SMILES SPONTANEOUSLY			CREEPS UPSTAIRS		
HEAD CONTROL			COOS AND CHUCKLES			SPEAKS 2 – 4 WORDS (OTHER THAN MAMA OR DADA), UNDERSTANDS MORE		
			RESPONDS TO SOUND					
MORO			RSA BY 6 MONTHS			LOOKS AT PICTURES, HELPS TURN PAGES		
ATNR			PULLED TO SITTING, HOLDS HEAD STEADILY			CASTS OBJECTS ON FLOOR REPEATEDLY		
			ROLLS BACK TO FRONT			TURNS HEAD TO SOUND		
LANDAU			PICKS UP OBJECT, SPOON OR 1 INCH CUBE, WHOLE HAND GRASP			RSA BY 18 - 20 MONTHS		
VISION SCREENING						WALKS UPSTAIRS WITH HELP		
HEARING SCREENING			BABBLES, E.G. REPEATS SOUNDS TOGETHER			POINTS TO PART OF BODY WHEN EXAMINER NAMES PART		
OVERALL DEVELOPMENT			HELD VERTICALLY WITH TOES TOUCHING, LEGS EXTENDED, KNEES LOCKED; NO SCISSORING					
						IMITATES HOUSEWORK		
CHRONOLOGICAL AGE			MORO DISAPPEARED			FEEDS SELF WITH SPOON		
			NO ANKLE CLONUS			TURNS 2 OR 3 PAGES AT ONCE		
ADJUSTED AGE			RESPONDS TO SOUND			TURNS HEAD TO SOUND		

PARENT – INFANT INTERACTION / FAMILY CONCERNS / ENVIRONMENT:

COPIES TO: ORIGINAL TO IDPH
PERINATAL CENTER
PUBLIC HEALTH NURSE
LOCAL PHYSICIAN

SIGNATURE _____

DATE _____

By permission of Illinois Department of Public Health.

114

REFERRAL CRITERIA AND PROCEDURE

Referral Criteria

I. Community Health Field Services of the Detroit Department of Health exist to improve the physical and emotional health status of the residents of Detroit. Public health nurses deliver comprehensive, individualized public health services in order to address specific health needs and concerns, modify health practices, give preventive and rehabilitative care, and promote ability for self-care. Health status assessment, health care instructions, counseling, problem solving, and referral service are available to specific individuals in their homes. The specific areas in which services are provided are maternal and child health, communicable disease, and developmental disability. No fees are charged for public health nursing services.

II. The following guidelines assist in the identification of individuals in need of a field referral:
   A. *Prenatal patients*—see Risk Scoring Index.* Refer all clients who score in the ultra high risk category.

   B. *Postpartum/neonatal*—see Risk Scoring Index*
   1. Refer all clients who score in the ultra high risk category.
   2. A baby with a birth weight of 3 lbs. 8 oz. (1,588 gm) or under is an automatic referral.

   C. Clients with developmental disabilities that occur before age 22 (for example, mental retardation).

   D. Crises (emergency situations).

Referral Procedure

I. Complete referral form (in triplicate).
   1. Complete all identifying data at top of form.
   2. List all pertinent information regarding problems.
   3. Action/outcome—list all outcomes as a result of action taken by you or your agency to assist client or resolve problem.
   4. Specify the nursing action requested.
      For example: Premature infant predischarge family assessment
         —Assess condition of infant, reinforce medical orders.
         —Review family support systems and resources.
         —Assess health needs and make appropriate referrals.
         —Parenting and infant care follow-up.
   5. Indicate whether reply is requested. If telephone reply is requested, indicate contact person and phone number.
   6. Hand deliver or mail two copies to Community Health Field Services; retain one copy for your record.

II. Additional information
   1. Written referral—allow 5 days for visit to be made. Allow an additional 2 weeks for form to be returned. Results of home visit can be returned by phone as soon as visit is made if requested.
   2. Telephone referrals—make a phone referral only for situations that require a visit within 24-48 hours.
   3. If you need or have additional information, please feel free to phone PHN or area supervisor.

* Scoring should be either prenatal or postnatal, not a combination of both.

MATERNAL - CHILD HEALTH RISK SCORING

Prenatal Index

1. Complete each category upon receipt of prenatal data.

2. Score identified conditions in each category.

3. Total each category.

4. Indicate grand total.

5. Refer all ultra high risk patients.

Grand total risk score key

0-3	Low risk
4-6	High risk
7+	Ultra high risk

Patient's name_____

Patient's number_____

Category 1
Maternal Factors

Social

Age ≤ 20 or ≥ 35	2	☐
Parity 0	1	☐
≥ 5	2	☐
Nonwhite	1	☐
Unmarried or no support system	1	☐
Education below 12th grade	1	☐
Low income	1	☐
Inappropriate behavior	1	☐

Past obstetric performance

Postpartum hemorrhage or third-stage problem	1	☐
Pregnancy termination	1	☐
Preeclampsia/hypertension	1	☐
Caesarean section	1	☐
Premature infant (1 or more)	1	☐
Stillborn/neonatal death	2	☐
Neurologically damaged infant	2	☐
Congential anomaly	2	☐
Prior Rh-affected infant	1	☐

Score____

Category 2
Associated conditions

Medical obstetric disorders

Renal disease	1	☐
Gestational diabetes	1	☐
Diabetes mellitus	2	☐
Heart disease	2	☐
Preeclampsia/toxemia	2	☐
Hypertension	2	☐
Endocrinopathy	2	☐
Infections	2	☐
Rh problem	2	☐
Other	1	☐

Nutrition

Obese	1	☐
Malnourished	1	☐
Anemia	1	☐

Substance abuse

Alcohol	2	☐
Drugs	2	☐
Tobacco	2	☐

Onset prenatal care

4-6 months	1	☐
7-9 months	2	☐

Score ____

Grand total ____

MATERNAL - CHILD HEALTH RISK SCORING

Postnatal Index

1. Complete each category upon receipt of prenatal data.

2. Score identified conditions in each category.

3. Total each category.

4. Indicate grand total.

5. Refer all ultra high risk patients.

Grand total risk score key

0-3	Low risk
4-6	High risk
7+	Ultra high risk

Patient's name_____

Patient's number_____

Category 1
Maternal Factors

Complications of labor and delivery

Bleeding	1	☐
Multiple births	2	☐
Breech or malpresentation	2	☐
Premature rupture of membranes	2	☐
Placenta previa	1	☐
Abruptio placentae	1	☐
Caesarean section	1	☐
Other	2	☐

Social factors

Age ≤ 20	2	☐
Unmarried	1	☐
Low income	1	☐
Education below 12th grade	1	☐
Nonwhite	1	☐
No prenatal care or third-trimester care only	2	☐
Fewer than 5 prenatal visits	1	☐

Associated conditions

Maternal illness	1	☐
Inappropriate behavior	2	☐
Substance abuse	2	☐
Unwanted baby	2	☐
Other	1	☐

Score____

Category 2
Neonatal factors

Neonatal factors

Gestation 37 weeks or less	2	☐
Gestation 42 weeks or more	2	☐
Weight 2,500 grams or less	2	☐
Weight 4,500 grams or more	2	☐
Apgar score 7 or less at 5 minutes	1	☐
ICU care—respiratory distress or hyaline membrane disease	2	☐
Meconium staining	1	☐
Fetal distress	1	☐
Drug-affected	1	☐
Congenital anomaly	2	☐
Birth injury	1	☐
Other	1	☐

Score ____

Grand total ____

MATERNAL-CHILD HEALTH RISK SCORING

Infant Index Ages 2-12 Months

1. Complete each category upon receipt of prenatal data.

2. Score identified conditions in each category.

3. Total each category.

4. Indicate grand total.

5. Refer all ultra high risk patients.

Automatic referral

1. Birth weight ≤ 1,588 grams ☐
   (3 lb. 8 oz.)

2. Developmental delay/disability ☐

Grand total risk score key

0-3 Low risk
4-6 High risk
7+ Ultra high risk

Patient's name _____

Patient's number _____

Category 1
Parental factors

Social

Mother ≤ age 20	2 ☐
Low income	1 ☐
Education below 12th grade	1 ☐
Nonwhite	1 ☐
No prenatal care or third-trimester care only	2 ☐
Unmarried or no support systems	2 ☐

Associated conditions

Substance abuse	2 ☐
Inappropriate behavior	2 ☐
Emotional or mental illness	2 ☐
Poor parenting skills	1 ☐
Chronic illness	1 ☐
Other	1 ☐

Score____

Category 2
Infant factors

Prematurity (≤ 37 weeks gestation)	2 ☐
Low birth weight (≤ 2,500 grams)	2 ☐
Prolonged hospitalization after birth	1 ☐
Congenital abnormality	2 ☐
Admissions to hospital for:	
Ingestions	2 ☐
Accidents	2 ☐
Respiratory conditions	1 ☐
Suspected child abuse/neglect	2 ☐
Failure to thrive	2 ☐
Other	1 ☐

Score ____

Grand total ____

By permission of Detroit Department of Public Health, Detroit, Michigan

PATIENT TRANSFER FORM

1. PHYSICIAN IN CHARGE AT TIME OF DISCHARGE	
2. WILL THIS PHYSICIAN CARE FOR PATIENT AFTER ADMISSION TO NEW FACILITY? YES NO	
3. FACILITY AND ADDRESS TRANSFERRING TO	ADDRESSOGRAPH STAMP

4. ADMITTED_____ DISCHARGED_____	5. HEALTH INSURANCE CLAIM NO.
6. FINAL DIAGNOSES	7. SURGICAL AND/OR MEDICAL PROCEDURES
8. ALLERGIES AND DRUG SENSITIVITIES	9. DOES PATIENT KNOW DIAGNOSES? YES_____ NO_____

10. DIET, DRUGS AND OTHER THERAPY AT TIME OF DISCHARGE (Not to be considered as admission orders)

11. (Check if present)

DISABILITIES	INCONTINENCE	IMPAIRMENTS	ACTIVITY TOLERANCE LIMITATIONS
☐ Amputation	☐ Bladder	☐ Mentality	☐ None
☐ Paralysis	☐ Bowel	☐ Speech	☐ Moderate
☐ Contracture	☐ Saliva	☐ Hearing	☐ Severe
☐ Decub. Ulcer		☐ Vision ☐ Sensation	

12. SELF CARE STATUS (Check one for each category)

A. FEEDING	Independent____	Needs Help_____	Cannot Feed Self_____
B. DRESSING	Independent____	Needs Help_____	Cannot Dress Self_____
C. ELIMINATION	Independent____	Help to Bathroom_____	Bedpan Required_____
D. BATHING	Independent____	Needs Help_____	Bed Bath with Help____ Bed Bath____
E. AMBULATORY STATUS	Independent____	Walks with Assistance_____	Bed Bound_____

13. MENTAL STATUS—COMMUNICATION ABILITY

A. Alert_____	E. Can write_____	I. Understands English_____
B. Forgetful_____	F. Understands speaking_____	(If no, state language spoken)
C. Confused_____	G. Understands writing_____	
D. Can speak_____	H. Understands gestures_____	_____

14. BEHAVIOR	15. PATIENT USES
Alcoholic_____ Suspicious_____	Colostomy_____ Catheter_____ Prosthesis_____
Senile_____ Noisy_____	Cane_____ Crutches_____ Walker_____
Belligerent_____ Withdrawn_____	Chair_____ Other_____

16. ADDITIONAL PERTINENT INFORMATION (Explain necessary details of care and treatment, including physical therapy requests)

Date_____   SIGNATURE_____

THE FOLLOWING COPIES HAVE BEEN MAILED TO:_____
                                                    (name of institution)

☐ H & P   ☐ X-ray_____   ☐ Admission Sheet   ☐ Other_____
                        (date)   (specify)

By permission of Georgia Baptist Medical Center, Atlanta, Georgia.

ADMISSION INFORMATION REFERRAL FORM

Patient's Name (Last, First, M.I.):	Date of Birth:	Sex:	Race:

Address For Care:	Social Security #:

Phone Number: ( )	Medicare #:

Directions:	Medicaid #:

	Other Insurance:

Dates of Stay in Hospital: From: To:	Date Plan Established:	Date Care to Start:

MEDICAL INFORMATION

Diagnosis:

Surgery Performed and Dates:

Allergies:	Diet:	Is Pt. informed of diagnosis? Yes ☐ No ☐

Home Health Services Needed:	Skilled Nursing ☐	Physical Therapy ☐	Occupational Therapy ☐	Speech Therapy ☐	Social Worker ☐	Home Health Aide ☐	Other (Specify) ☐

Activity:

Orders For Patient Care:

_____

_____

_____

_____

_____

_____

Additional Information:

_____

☐ CERTIFICATION ☐ RECERTIFICATION: I certify that the above named patient (1) is under my care, (2) is homebound except when receiving outpatient services, (3) requires skilled nursing care on an intermittent basis or physical or speech therapy as specified in the original orders with the modifications listed above.

Referring Physician: _____

Signature: _____

Name: _____

Address: _____

_____

Phone: _____

Discharge Planning Nurse:

Signature: _____

Phone: _____

Date: _____

By permission of Georgia Baptist Medical Center, Atlanta, Georgia.

AMBULANCE TRANSPORT FORM

_____

Patient Name: _____ Date: _____

Destination From: **Georgia Baptist Medical Center** Room: _____

To: _____ Return: _____

Medicare #: _____ Medicaid #: _____

Age: _____ Date of Birth: _____

Doctor's Name: _____ Address: _____

Phone: _____ _____

Diagnosis: _____

_____

_____

Person Responsible: _____ Address: _____

                                          _____
                                                                        (zip)

Due to patient's diagnosis and condition, it is medically necessary
that the patient be transported by ambulance.

_____ (Doctor)

_____ (Nurse)

                                          Date: _____

By permission of Georgia Baptist Medical Center, Atlanta, Georgia.

POSTHOSPITAL CARE PLAN: HEART FAILURE

When the heart has difficulty pumping enough blood to the body tissues it is said to have failed. Most heart failure will respond to treatment, but the degree of success varies in different people. Treatment of heart failure requires your active cooperation with activity, diet and medication.

Activity: You can help your heart by getting enough rest and following a sensible activity/exercise schedule. Ask your doctor what kind of activity or exercise is best for you.
- Plan your day so you don't exhaust yourself.
- Do only one thing at a time and rest awhile before doing the next.
- When you are awake don't stay in any one position longer than one hour. When you sit down, try to put your feet up. Try not to cross your legs or ankles.
- Ask your doctor if you may climb stairs.
ADDITIONAL INSTRUCTIONS:

Diet: A proper diet, involving weight control and a mild restriction of sodium (salt) and cholesterol, is an important part of your treatment. Medical research has shown that the following two conditions, along with excessive weight, increase the risk of heart failure:
    1.) a high salt intake can cause your body to hold extra fluids,
    2.) dietary cholesterol (a type of animal fat) can build up on the walls of the heart's blood vessels.
- If you are overweight, lose the amount of weight recommended by your doctor or dietitian.
- Avoid overeating at meal-times, as this causes a greater work effort by the heart in digesting the excessive food.
- All your foods should be prepared and eaten without salt (this includes garlic, onion and celery salts).
- Avoid "salty" foods such as peanuts, potato chips, ham, bacon, luncheon meats, soups, salad dressings, pickles, mustard, catsup, etc.
- Avoid food prepared with breading, stuffing, cream sauces and gravy.
- Whenever possible, use FRESH foods rather than canned or frozen.
- Do not drink softened water; (bottled distilled water or "Chicago" water are good substitutes).
- Salt substitutes and alcoholic beverages are allowed only with your doctor's permission.
- Avoid foods high in cholesterol and high in saturated (animal) fat.
- Replace a great percentage of the "saturated" (animal) fat with "polyunsaturated" (vegetable) fat.
- Eat fish, poultry and veal more often than beef, lamb or pork.
- Eat less organ meats such as liver.
- Use vegetable oil (polyunsaturate) margarine and skim or lowfat milk.
- Limit eggs to 3 a week.
- Eat fewer commercial, baked and frozen foods containing whole milk, butter and eggs.
Your doctor or you may request the dietitian to instruct you further in the details of this diet.

MEDICATION:

Your medicine is intended to help increase the efficiency of your heart. It is important that you take all your medicine exactly as prescribed.
- Do not change the amount of medicine you take, or stop taking any medicine unless your doctor tells you to do so.
- Do not take any medicine unless you discuss it with your doctor. This includes laxatives, vitamins, cold tablets, or arthritis preparations.

When having your prescriptions filled, ask your pharmacist to help you complete this section.

NAME	DESCRIPTION	TIME
-------------------	-------------------	-------------------
-------------------	-------------------	-------------------
-------------------	-------------------	-------------------
-------------------	-------------------	-------------------
-------------------	-------------------	-------------------

PERSONAL HYGIENE:

It is important that you:
- Weigh yourself at the same time every morning. (Do this after you urinate and before you eat breakfast. Be sure that you are always either nude or wearing the same type of clothing). Record the weight in a diary or on a calender. Take the record with you each time you see your doctor.
- Don't wear panty girdles or round garters. Avoid similiar types of clothing that restrict your circulation in one area.
- Bathe or shower as before you got sick, but avoid very hot or very cold water.
- Don't use a heating pad unless you discuss this with your doctor.

ADDITIONAL INSTRUCTIONS:

FOLLOW UP CARE:

Control of your problem depends a great deal on how well you follow your physician's advice. Make an appointment to see your doctor within two weeks after you leave the hospital.

It is also important that you call your doctor if you:
- Gain more than 3 pounds in 2 days.
- Feel more tired or weak than usual.
- If you have trouble breathing, especially at night or need more pillows than usual to breathe easy when you are lying down.
- Cough more than usual.
- You have to urinate more often during the night.
- Have a temperature.
- Have no appetite, nausea or vomiting that lasts more than one day.

ADDITIONAL INSTRUCTIONS:

By permission of Little Company of Mary Hospital, Evergreen Park, Illinois.

JOB DESCRIPTION

Discharge Planning Coordinator

FUNCTION

The discharge planning coordinator organizes the discharge planning program and recommends policies and procedures to provide a planned program of continuing care that meets patients' postdischarge needs.

RESPONSIBILITY

The Medical Center delegates the responsibility for the execution of the discharge planning program to the discharge planning coordinator.

QUALIFICATIONS

Education

Graduate of an accredited school of nursing.

Registered and currently licensed in the state.

A masters degree in a health-related field.

Personal Characteristics

Capacity to relate well to patients and their families, as well as to hospital personnel.

Leadership ability and ability to motivate others.

Ability to gain the respect of the medical staff and administration.

Job Knowledge and Experience

Experience in an administrative position.

Familiarity with all aspects of patient care.

Experience in community health, home care, or discharge planning.

Familiarity with the organization and functions of related departments in the hospital.

Knowledge of follow-up regimens and home care theory.

Familiarity with community resources and government programs.

DUTIES

1. Recommends goals and objectives for the department with projected deadlines, means of effecting changes, and an evaluative system for assessing results.
2. Evaluates the discharge planning system on an ongoing basis, researches methods of improvement and ways of implementing change.
3. Serves as a consultant to departments involved in the discharge planning process.
4. Monitors discharge planning activities of various departments. Suggests corrective action where appropriate
5. Monitors appropriateness of individual discharge plans.
6. Monitors documentation of individual discharge plans.
7. Conducts and participates in educational programs related to discharge planning for hospital staff.
8. Participates in appropriate meetings and serves as an active member on appropriate committees, such as the utilization review committee.
9. Establishes and maintains liaison with local community resources.
10. Provides statistical data to administration.

JOB DESCRIPTION

Discharge Planning Nurse

QUALIFICATIONS

Education

Graduate of an accredited school of nursing.

Registered and currently licensed in the state.

A bachelor of science degree or equivalent experience.

Personal Characteristics

Demonstrated capacity to relate well to patients and their families and hospital personnel.

Leadership ability and ability to motivate others.

Ability to gain the respect of the medical staff.

Job Knowledge and Experience

Familiarity with all aspects of patient care.

Experience in supervisory positions.

Familiarity with the organization and functions of the related departments in the hospital.

Knowledge of follow-up regimens and home care theory.

Familiarity with community resources and government programs.

DUTIES

1. Provides discharge planning assessments on all patients identified to the department as requiring services. Documents on patient's charts.
2. Conducts interdisciplinary patient rounds on the units on a regular basis. Keeps a record of discharge plans, health team involvement, and possible action necessary.
3. Recommends appropriate discharge plans to the health team.
4. Reviews patient's chart and interviews patient and family when the involvement of the discharge planner seems indicated.
5. Confers with physician and health team members as indicated.
6. Makes referrals to appropriate departments.
7. Encourages adequate documentation of the discharge plan on patient charts.

POSITION DESCRIPTION

Liaison Nurse for Discharge Planning

DEFINITION

The liaison nurse for discharge planning is a registered nurse who helps with plans for the discharge of a patient from the hospital to the home, or to another care facility.

QUALIFICATIONS

Professional

Graduation from an accredited school of nursing and current licensure.

At least a year's experience as a staff nurse; head nurse experience desirable.

Active participation in the professional nursing organizations.

Continuing education in the field of discharge planning.

Personal

Good health and grooming.

Emotional stability.

Initiative and determination.

Integrity.

Good judgment.

A friendly, understanding attitude.

Good interpersonal relationships.

FUNCTIONS

Plans for use of resources within the community that supplement and reinforce the discharge planning activities of the hospital.

Assists the nursing staff, physicians, other hospital personnel, and the patient's family to become better prepared in evaluating patient care needs and planning for continuing care of patients after their discharge from the hospital.

Orients patient and family for the purpose of transfer.

Continues to coordinate the stages between illness and recovery, long-term and short-term.

Assesses patient's needs, stimulates and redirects his thinking, and encourages self-expression, self-evaluation, and self-determination.

Provides information to the patient, by teaching and demonstration, using all available resources.

Acquaints the medical staff, nursing staff, and other health professionals with the discharge planning program, meets with them at intervals to explain and inform.

Meets with public health and social service personnel.

Makes rounds to all nursing units on a daily basis to review discharge plans. Participates in team conferences on units.

Discusses discharge plan with physician and obtains necessary orders for referral.

Makes notations on patient's Kardex or chart when problems are noted.

Attends monthly meetings of audit utilization committee.

Keeps statistical records of activities and referrals.

Turns in monthly to director of nursing and administrator a report on hospital stay and discharge plans on those patients for whom she provides help.

JOB SUMMARY

Function cooperatively with social service to plan and coordinate planning for posthospital care. Meet regularly to review all pending and new referrals and available community resources.

Work primarily on the nursing units to identify and assess patient needs for continuity of care.

Plan with the nursing personnel for patient/family teaching in preparation for discharge.

Counsel with the patient/family in planning for patient care and rehabilitative measures in the home situation as early as possible.

Make rounds to all nursing units daily to review discharge plans and make progress notes on patient's chart to keep physician informed of the progress and details of the planning.

Discuss discharge plans with physicians to obtain necessary orders for referrals.

Review admissions daily (or as soon after admission as possible) to initially evaluate a patient's need for discharge planning.

Consult with other allied health personnel within the hospital (such as physical therapist, dietitian, etc.) whose assistance is essential in planning for optimum continuity of care after discharge.

Participate in team conferences on nursing units to discuss the discharge planning process; to assess a patient's needs for continuity of care, to develop a plan for care after discharge from the hospital; to determine ways to implement the plan of care and to emphasize the value of the team approach in giving total patient care.

Make referrals to the area public health departments and other agencies as indicated. Complete necessary referral forms to convey adequate and accurate information regarding the patient to the health agency.

Maintain accurate records and keep copies of referrals on file for future reference.

Participate in the orientation of nursing personnel and work in cooperation with the inservice department in explaining and teaching the concepts of continuity of care and discharge planning.

Work in cooperation with social service and the utilization review committee in ensuring the proper utilization of hospital beds.

By permission of Emmett Memorial Hospital, Clifton Forge, Virginia.

POSITION DESCRIPTION

Discharge Planning Coordinator (VNA)

PRIMARY PURPOSE OF POSITION

To assist hospital and nursing home staffs in assessing patients' needs in order to ensure continuity of care at the appropriate level upon discharge.

QUALIFICATIONS

Licensure: Current licensure or eligibility for licensure as a registered nurse.
Education: Baccalaureate degree in nursing from a college or university with an accredited National League for Nursing program.
Experience: Two years' experience in community health nursing under supervision.

OR

Education: Graduation from a National League for Nursing or state-approved school of nursing.
Experience: Four years' experience with two years in community health nursing under supervision.

DUTIES AND RESPONSIBILITIES

Responsible to executive director.

Establishes contact with appropriate hospital and nursing home personnel to interpret discharge planning services available.

Is knowledgeable of community resources in order that appropriate utilization and referrals may be implemented for the benefit of the patient.

Confers with patients, families, and hospital staff in order to assess needs at time of discharge.

When deemed necessary, arranges for a visit to patient's home to determine potential for home care.

Visits and obtains progress reports on inpatients for whom the agency has been providing service, in order to ensure continuity of care.

Provides information to agency regarding potential referrals and plans of treatment.

Keeps executive director informed of community contacts and maintains system of records and reports.

Works with educational director in planning inservice education and orientation of new personnel in the area of discharge planning.

Participates in agency's program for student experiences.

As a representative of the agency, participates and plans with other community agencies and physicians in their efforts to ensure continuity of care.

Participates actively in her professional nursing organization.

By permission of Instructive Visiting Nurse Association, Richmond, Virginia.

DISCHARGE PLANNING COORDINATOR

Performance Description

TITLE: *Discharge planning coordinator*　　　　　DIVISION: *Administration*

RESPONSIBLE TO: *Chief executive officer, Center Hospital*

PURPOSE: To design, implement and continuously evaluate a planned program of continuing care that will meet the postdischarge needs of the patients.

PERFORMANCE RESPONSIBILITIES	PERFORMANCE IS SATISFACTORY WHEN
1. *To Chief Executive Officer*	
1.1. Function within the philosophy and policies of Center Hospital.	1.1. Support of the philosophy and policies is evidenced through both written and oral expression.
1.2. Design and assist in the development of the discharge planning program. Coordinate the program's daily operation.	1.2. Discharge planning activities focus on the achievement/sustainment of desired patient care outcomes.
1.3. Supervise and evaluate discharge planning activities.	1.3. Review and evaluation of the appropriateness and effectiveness of discharge planning activities are in progress.
1.4. Develop methods/systems for the documentation of discharge planning activities/functions.	1.4. Documentation substantiates the existence and effectiveness of the discharge planning program.
1.5. Chair the discharge planning committee.	1.5. Discharge planning plans/problems are reviewed/discussed/investigated. Recommendations for program development and problem resolution are communicated to appropriate personnel. Recommendations enhance/facilitate program development.
1.6. Seek assistance from chief executive officer as necessary and appropriate.	1.6. Specific instances of seeking and using such help occur.
1.7. Facilitate the process of change.	1.7. Desired change takes place.
1.8. Participate in utilization review and quality assurance studies as appropriate.	1.8. Data is properly collected. Pertinent findings are applied/implemented.
2. *To Patients and Families*	
2.1. Patients' needs are assessed. Self-expression, self-evaluation, and self-determination are encouraged.	2.1. Discharge plan reflects patients' input.
2.2. Confer with patient and family members to assess their plans/desires/understanding.	2.2. Such meetings take place and reflect good communication.
2.3. Provide information for patient and family by teaching, demonstration, or other appropriate techniques.	2.3. Patient and family demonstrate knowledge of plan and rationale for actions.
2.4. Discuss method of transfer and any unusual arrangements with patient and family.	2.4. Patient and family can describe all components of discharge plan.

PERFORMANCE RESPONSIBILITIES	PERFORMANCE IS SATISFACTORY WHEN
3. *To Nursing Department*	
3.1. Functions as consultant in all matters related to patient discharge planning.	3.1. Assistance, provided as necessary or requested, facilitates the discharge planning process.
3.2. Makes daily rounds on all nursing units to review discharge plans and participate in problem solving related to posthospital care planning.	3.2. Such rounds are made. Problems are referred to appropriate sources for resolution.
3.3. Coordinate input from nursing staff to evaluate and improve discharge planning activities.	3.3. Staff input is solicited and utilized to develop innovative and comprehensive discharge planning activities.
4. *To Other Professionals and Organizations*	
4.1. Maintains positive relationships with members of other health care disciplines.	4.1. Feedback is positive and purpose of communication is achieved.
4.2. Assists other health care personnel to improve their evaluation of patient care needs and planning for posthospital care.	4.2. Patients' posthospital plans of care reflect input of knowledgeable health professionals.
4.3. Identifies community resources. Participates in professional organizations as appropriate and necessary.	4.3. Community resources are utilized to supplement and reinforce the hospital's discharge planning activities.
5. *To Self*	
5.1. Maintains sense of personal satisfaction; keeps knowledge and skills current.	5.1. Personal goals are met as related to job performance.
5.2. Participates in educational activities.	5.2. New learning provides sense of growth and development.

QUALIFICATIONS

1. Currently licensed as a registered professional nurse in state.

2. Bachelor's degree required. Master's degree preferred.

3. Minimum of three years' experience in discharge planning, public health, or home health care.

4. Ability to work well with a diverse group of health care professionals.

5. Leadership ability and the ability to motivate others.

6. Demonstrated skills in writing, communication, and interpersonal relationships.

7. Familiarity with community resources and government programs.

The authors wish to acknowledge the work of Warren and Joan Ganong on performance appraisal. Their early writings in the *Ganong Newsletter* provided the initial ideas that formed the basis for the development of this, and many other, performance descriptions.

QUALITY ASSURANCE PROCESS

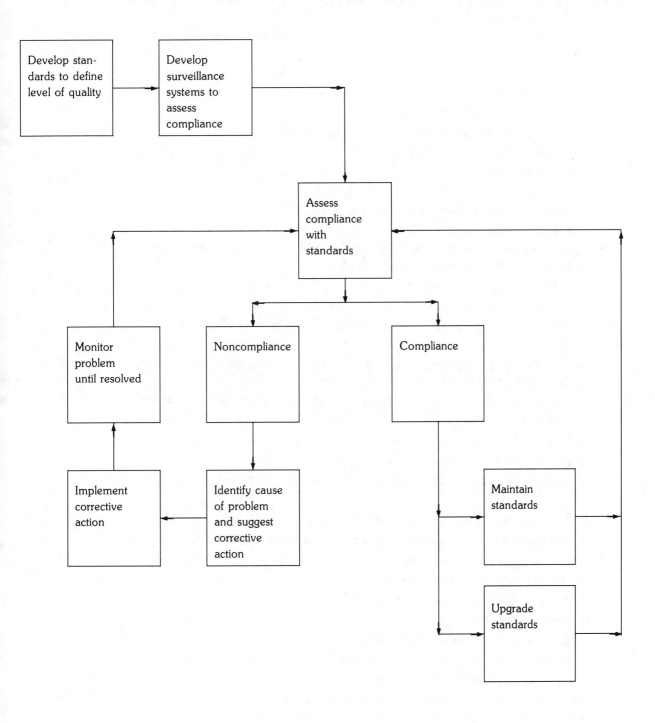

DISCHARGE PLANNING PROGRAM
EVALUATION TOOL

by Garnett Jones, RN

1	2	3	4

I. Patients with discharge planning needs are identified and planning is initiated as early as is feasible:

A. The operation of the admissions department includes activities that initiate discharge planning:

    1. Information is collected during the preadmission/admission process regarding:

        a. Expected length of stay.

        b. Plans for care after discharge.

        c. Anticipated problems related to care after discharge.

    2. Information relative to discharge planning is provided to the discharge planning department daily:

        a. Copies of face sheets of all new admissions.

        b. List of new admissions, including diagnoses.

        c. List of new patients identified by high-risk criteria.

B. Activities within the discharge planning department facilitate the identification of patients with potential postdischarge care needs:

    1. Review of face sheets daily.

    2. Review of patient lists daily.

    3. Review of patients on each unit (Kardex rounds) at least weekly.

    4. Department maintains visibility and availability.

C. The initial nursing assessment completed at the time of admission includes collection of data that identifies discharge planning problems:

    1. Patient's perception of own health status, treatment regimen, and care needs.

    2. Present living arrangements.

    3. Psychosocial and economic status.

    4. Patient's plans for care after discharge.

    5. Self-care deficits related to the illness or to resource limitations:

        a. Current.

        b. Anticipated, related to diagnoses and treatment plans.

    6. Family's perception of patient's needs and plans for care after discharge.

D. The nursing care plan written after the initial nursing assessment includes the following:

    1. Description of present living arrangements.

    2. Tentative plans for care after discharge.

    3. Discharge planning problems:

        a. Self-care deficits related to illness or injury.

        b. Self-care deficits related to resource limitations.

    4. Planned interventions related to problems.

E. Identified patients with discharge planning problems are referred to appropriate team members or discharge planning department in a timely manner:

    1. Nursing staffs refers patients at the time of the initial nursing assessment, or as soon as the needs are identified.

Key: 1 = 86-100% occurrence
      2 = 51- 85% occurrence
      3 = 26- 50% occurrence
      4 = 1- 25% occurrence

1	2	3	4

2. Physicians refer patients as soon as needs are identified and do not wait until just before discharge.

3. Other team members refer patients at the time of their initial assessments, or when needs are identified.

4. Utilization review staff refer patients at the time of the first review, or as soon as problems are identified.

F. Health care providers in the community contact the discharge planning department in a timely manner regarding anticipated problems with postdischarge care of patients recently admitted.

II. Patients have access to assistance with discharge planning:

A. The referral system facilitates the timely referral of patients with discharge planning needs to the appropriate team members:

1. Patients and families may refer themselves to the discharge planning department for assistance without a physician's order.

2. Health team members may refer a patient to the discharge planning department without a physician's order.

3. Discharge planning staff may assess for needs and begin to develop a tentative plan for postdischarge care without a physician's order.

4. The mechanism by which referrals are made is simple and may be accomplished quickly.

B. Discharge planning staff are available to patients, families, physicians, and other team members, including community health care providers:

1. The ratio of staff to patient population and case mix is adequate to meet the needs of the patients and the program.

2. The staff is located on site and provides ready availability.

3. Coverage is provided full time, and may include evenings and weekends as needed.

III. The discharge planning is centralized:

A. One person is designated to be responsible and accountable for the discharge planning program.

B. There is a policy and mechanism for referring patients to the discharge planning department.

C. There is a discharge planning committee made up of representatives from predominant disciplines and departments.

IV. The discharge planning program is multidisciplinary:

A. Nursing assesses for discharge planning needs and initiates action by intervention and referral.

B. Social services actively participates in discharge planning by assisting all other disciplines as needed.

C. The following ancillary disciplines actively participate:

1. Dietary.

2. Physical therapy.

3. Respiratory therapy.

4. Occupational therapy.

5. Speech therapy.

6. Clinical nursing specialists.

7. Chaplains.

8. Patient advocates.

9. Others.

1	2	3	4

V. The discharge planning program is coordinated:

A. Patient rounds include all involved disciplines.

B. Pre-discharge planning conferences are attended by all involved disciplines.

C. Predominant disciplines are represented on the discharge planning committee.

D. All involved disciplines document their discharge planning activities, including a discharge summary in the patient's record.

E. The nursing care plan indicates involvement by other disciplines.

F. The discharge planning coordinator is a member of the utilization review committee.

G. The discharge planning coordinator is a member of the quality assurance committee.

VI. The discharge planning program is individualized and patient centered:

A. The initial nursing assessment is comprehensive and holistic in approach.

B. Goals for care after discharge are mutually set with the patient and his significant others.

C. Interventions are planned and adapted to needs specific to the individual patient, taking into consideration the patient's resources, preferences, life-style, and abilities.

D. All team members use a holistic approach when providing discharge planning assistance.

E. The patient is provided with complete information about alternative care plans that may be available and is allowed to make choices and decisions in developing a final plan.

VII. Documentation is an integral part of the process:

A. There is a common source document for all discharge planning activities.

B. Notes made in locations other than the patient's medical record are cross-referenced in the patient's medical record.

C. Documentation occurs:

    1. When activity takes place.

    2. At least every 7 days when there is long-term involvement.

D. Documentation is:

    1. Identifiable as to name, discipline, and telephone number of person entering.

    2. Specific, denoting levels of care, patient needs, names of agencies, vendors, caregivers, etc.

E. Documentation shows:

    1. Knowledge and involvement of patient and his significant others.

    2. Involvement of physicians.

    3. Interdisciplinary communication when applicable.

F. Discharge summary information is:

    1. Documented in the patient's medical record:

        a. On common source document *or*

        b. Nursing discharge summary *or*

        c. Multidisciplinary discharge summary.

    2. Provided to those responsible for next level of care:

        a. Other inpatient facility.

        b. Home health agency.

        c. Physician.

        d. Patient and significant other.

    3. Maintained in the patient's medical record as a copy of referral information sent to next provider of care when indicated.

VIII. Education is a part of the discharge planning program:

	1	2	3	4

    A. The coordinator participates in orientation of new personnel, including physicians, on a regular basis.

    B. The coordinator meets with various disciplines on a regular basis, especially nursing, to keep them current regarding the discharge planning program.

    C. Students from various professional health care disciplines matriculate through the department to learn about discharge planning coordination.

    D. The department interacts with the community to promote mutual understanding of continuity of care needs.

IX. An evaluation mechanism is an integral part of the ongoing process:

    A. Standards of practice are defined and adopted for the program:

        1. Structure.

        2. Process.

        3. Outcome.

    B. Audits are conducted:

        1. Scheduled audits.

        2. Requested audits.

        3. Designated audits.

    C. Practical methods for collecting evaluation data are adopted:

        1. Patient questionnaires.

        2. Community agency questionnaires.

        3. Patient surveys by telephone.

        4. Data collection via reporting mechanisms of professional staff.

2591-N-860106
5-18